WHY
INFANT
REFLUX
MATTERS

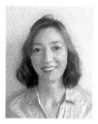

About the author

Carol Smyth is an IBCLC (International Board Certified Lactation Consultant) working in a busy private practice in Northern Ireland. She became interested in babies and reflux when her first son was diagnosed and treated for reflux in his early weeks. After receiving breastfeeding support and learning more about brain development, she realised that many of the symptoms that had been diagnosed as reflux had either been misinterpreted or were resolved by small changes in care. This revelation inspired her to change career and retrain as an IBCLC.

Within her private practice she is driven by a passion to minimise the gap between our understanding of normal baby behaviours and societal norms through education and supporting parents. Understanding the level of anxious distress parents can feel when they have an unsettled baby, and with a background in psychology, she uses CBT techniques and education to lower anxiety alongside practical strategies to reduce reflux.

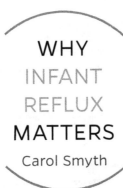

WHY
INFANT
REFLUX
MATTERS

Carol Smyth

pinter
&
martin

Why Infant Reflux Matters (Pinter & Martin Why It Matters 21)

First published by Pinter & Martin Ltd 2021, reprinted 2024

©2021 Carol Smyth

ISBN 978-1-78066-640-2

Also available as an ebook

Pinter & Martin Why It Matters ISSN 2056-8657

Series editor: Susan Last
Index: Helen Bilton
Cover Design: Blok Graphic, London
Cover Illustration: Lucy Davey
Illustrations: Salma Price-Nell at thesalsacreative.com
Author photograph: Will Smyth

British Library Cataloguing-in-Publication Data
A catalogue record for this book is available from the British Library.

Set in Minion

This book has been printed on paper that is sourced and harvested from sustainable forests and is FSC accredited.

Pinter & Martin Ltd
Unit 803 Omega Works
4 Roach Road
London E3 2PH

pinterandmartin.com

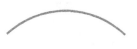

Contents

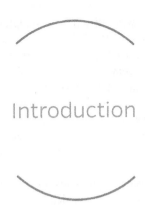

Introduction

The diagnosis of gastro-oesophageal reflux disease (GORD) in babies has skyrocketed in the last 25 years, with studies suggesting that as many as 1 in 20 babies in many countries may be on medication for GORD. If you, as a parent, do an internet search for symptoms of reflux or GORD you might find any of the following symptoms listed:

- Spitting up
- Feeding difficulties (e.g. gagging, choking, refusing feeds)
- Hiccups or coughing
- Fussiness/crying/irritability
- Arching the back
- Seems to be in pain/distressed behaviour
- Weight gain issues (low or high weight gain)
- Colicky or windy
- Clingy/sensitive
- Poor sleep/frequent waking
- Doesn't like to lie on back

The problem with this list of symptoms is that they are general. Many of the behaviours listed above are also symptomatic of a feeding or baby care issue. In fact these symptoms more usually indicate a fixable feeding or baby care problem rather than a problem with a baby's stomach acid production. Some of them are also normal, expected, but misunderstood behaviours in young babies.

In my experience (and in the experience of many of my colleagues), many babies with the symptoms above are placed on a trial of reflux medications before feeding is adequately assessed, and feeding problems or misinterpretations of normal behaviour have been ruled out. Every drug has side-effects, and in my experience most parents would rather find solutions which do not involve giving their baby medications at a young age. This book can help you work through the causes of reflux and find the reason for your baby's symptoms and practical solutions in order to reduce or eliminate them without medication.

My experience with reflux and feeding babies

When I had my first baby I knew little of infant reflux. I was perhaps a little naive in my understanding of normal baby behaviour and my expectations were culturally based (I thought my baby would feed every three hours and sleep in his crib in between). Confronted with a baby who fed every two hours and wanted to be held on my body almost all the time made me feel anxious and concerned. He just didn't want to sleep, or be, anywhere else. When he was just three weeks old I went to a breastfeeding support group hosted by the local community nursing team. I drove to the group with my baby in his car seat. He was still asleep when I arrived and I carried the car seat into the group. An hour later he was still asleep. Since he never usually slept this long without being held I mentioned it to the nurses. One of them suggested that since he was sleeping longer in the car seat, perhaps he had reflux. I went home and started to research reflux on the internet, only to find that I could fit his need to be with me, his high weight gain, his frequent waking and not wanting to be laid down on his back into a possible reflux diagnosis. At our six-week doctor checkup I laid him down on the examination bed to unbutton his babygro and he cried. I picked him up as I wriggled his clothes off and he immediately snuggled into me and stopped crying. I laid him down to undo his nappy and he cried. I took the nappy off, lifted him up to my shoulder and he stopped crying. My doctor then remarked, 'I see that he cries when you leave him down. He may have a bit of reflux'. To me, that was a diagnosis. Within a couple of weeks my baby was on medication. I felt trapped. I didn't want to give him the medication, but I also didn't want my baby to be in pain.

That was the start of my journey into learning about babies, nervous system development, feeding and reflux. With some support around feeding I learned that my baby did not actually have reflux, but that his symptoms were actually behaviours that I didn't understand. This sparked a passion in me around resolving feeding issues and I quickly trained to become a breastfeeding counsellor and later to qualify as an IBCLC (International Board Certified Lactation Consultant). Through my training to become an IBCLC I learned about physiologically normal feeding behaviours and patterns, and as I worked with babies and parents I realised that the symptoms that are often misdiagnosed as reflux in breastfed babies are also common in babies being fed with bottles. I developed a special interest in helping families dealing with (or querying) reflux, and helping them to resolve the problems by looking at the wider feeding and infant development picture: frequency of feeds, volume in each feed, latch to breast/bottle, swallowing pattern, reading baby's behavioural cues, understanding infant nervous system needs and so on. I now have a private practice as well as workshops and webinars helping parents and educating other health professionals.

How to use this book

The book is written in two parts. The first part reviews what we know about reflux so far: what reflux is and what it isn't; the difference between reflux and GORD (gastro-oesophageal reflux disease); and what research says about normal physiology. It will cover our cultural norms and how they may differ from what is physiologically normal for a baby's digestion. It will discuss the societal pressures on parents which may also contribute to reflux symptoms. It will probe the role of acid in a baby's digestion, what happens if that acid is suppressed and also look at what the research suggests about whether reflux in babies causes pain due to acid burning the oesophagus. It will look at the current common treatment pattern and the effect it has on the body and empower you as a parent to make informed choices about your baby's feeding.

The second part is designed to help you work through the causes of symptoms that are commonly attributed to reflux and ways of altering feeding and feeding patterns which may alleviate those symptoms. Some of you will be breastfeeding and some will be feeding by bottle (whether that is expressed breastmilk or infant formula milk), and there are specific areas for each under each symptom and specific solutions for each method of feeding. Part two also identifies symptoms which should be looked at by a healthcare professional and possible treatments to normalise feeding. It also includes the stories of real babies that I have worked with, so that you can see how these solutions work in the real world.

I think that most parents want to help their baby to thrive without medication, if they can possibly avoid it. My aim in this book is to help you to do that, and to understand a little more about your baby along the way.

PART I

What is Reflux?

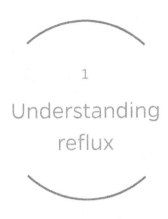

1

Understanding reflux

What is reflux (GOR)?

Reflux, technically known as gastro-oesophageal reflux (GOR), is considered to be the movement of the stomach contents from the stomach into the oesophagus. Reflux is considered to be normal in babies. The stomach contents may come out of the baby's mouth (spitting up), or may not. In US English it may be referred to as gastro-esophageal reflux. Note the slightly different spelling and that the acronym becomes GER rather than GOR. In this book I will use the UK English spelling, but the terms mean exactly the same thing.

The volume of milk that a baby may spit up can vary widely between babies. Some babies may spit up a little after each feed, often referred to as 'posseting'. Other babies spit up large amounts after each feed. It can seem as though they are spitting up whole feeds, causing a lot of anxiety for parents about how much milk they are keeping down, and it can require multiple daily changes of clothes for both baby and caregiver. Most babies with reflux are somewhere in between, perhaps spitting up after some feeds but not all, and are unconcerned by the spit up (even if the parent/caregiver is). In other babies the reflux

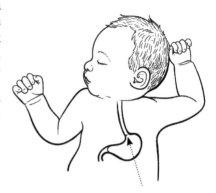

Figure 1: Location of the lower oesophageal sphincter (LOS)

may not reach the mouth. It may move out of the stomach, travel partly up the oesophagus and then return to the stomach, or it may reach the mouth but be re-swallowed. This is often referred to as 'silent reflux', or in some texts as 'occult regurgitation'. Silent reflux is again considered to be normal in babies and in most babies there is little outward sign that the reflux has happened.

Why does reflux happen?

We can consider a baby's stomach to be like a bag which holds the milk that a baby drinks. The top and the bottom of the stomach have valves which can open or close in order to hold the contents inside or let them out. The valve at the top of the stomach is called the lower oesophageal sphincter (LOS) and consists of a series of muscles and tissue. The muscles can contract and close the valve, or relax and allow the valve to open. In US English this is referred to as the LES (lower esophageal sphincter). When a baby sucks and swallows, the swallow triggers the LOS to relax and open in order to allow the swallowed milk to enter the stomach. The LOS muscles then contract and close the valve to the stomach again. When there is repeated swallowing, as a breastfed baby would during a milk ejection (also known as a letdown), or a bottle-fed baby does with a fast teat flow, the LOS remains relaxed and open until after the last swallow, and only then contracts to close the stomach.[1] Milk then remains in the stomach and digestion begins, via the stomach acid. Once chemical digestion has reached the required level, the valve at the bottom of the stomach (the pyloric sphincter) opens and the stomach contents move into the intestines for further digestion. Breastmilk empties from the stomach in around 45 minutes, infant formula in about 75 minutes.[2]

The LOS doesn't only relax with a swallow. It also relaxes at other times without being triggered by a swallow, and these openings are called TLOSRs (transient lower oesophageal sphincter relaxations). These transient relaxations or openings of the sphincter muscle are triggered either from the stomach or from the throat.

The vast majority of TLOSR openings are triggered from the stomach, at times when the stomach is stretched or distended. This distension can happen because of the volume of food that we eat or drink. The stretching of the stomach triggers TLOSRs so that excess food or liquid can escape. We can think of this opening in the same way as an overflow in a bath or sink, which allows excess water to escape safely. This is essentially a safety or comfort mechanism which allows a baby who has drunk too much milk to get rid of the excess.

In addition, when we swallow, we may take in a little air, particularly if we are gulping and rushing the meal. As we continue to swallow throughout the course of a meal or drink we build up the amount of air in the stomach. A crying baby may also swallow air while crying. This air distends the stomach and triggers the safety TLOSR mechanism. The LOS opens in order to let the air move back up into the oesophagus and escape through the mouth and nose. This happens to us frequently each day without us being aware of it. In other words, if the stomach becomes overfull, either of milk or through air swallowed along with the milk, then the overflow valve opens in order to regulate the level of food and gas in the stomach.

A smaller number of TLOSR openings come from the throat. Above we discussed how a swallow triggers the opening of the stomach valve, but it seems that small contractions in the throat can also trigger TLOSR openings. These may be considered incomplete or partial swallows. This will be relevant in later chapters when we look at the 'suck, swallow, breathe' mechanism in babies and what can affect it. A further cause of TLOSR is increased abdominal pressure, through abdominal straining, coughing, raising legs, crying, and passing stools. This is significant as it can be easy to interpret a crying baby as being sore due to reflux, when it may be that the reflux is caused by the crying.

Positioning and muscle tone also play a role. As adults we are upright most of the time and so reflux of stomach contents has to happen against gravity. A TLOSR which happens in an adult in order to release some gas is unlikely to cause the adult to vomit. Young babies, however, are only upright if held upright. They do not yet have the neuromuscular control which allows them to sit or stand and so they often spend much of their time lying down or reclined, meaning that the oesophagus is often horizontal, or semi-horizontal, allowing a much easier outflow of stomach contents if a TLOSR does happen.

It may be that some babies also have lower tone in their LOS, meaning that it is always more relaxed than in other babies, and therefore more reflux is present. This may be why some babies spit up frequently, while others rarely do.

What is considered normal?

Since feeding often causes the stomach to stretch or have increased pressure, and we know that stretching or increased pressure causes TLOSRs, reflux is considered to be an entirely normal physiological process of a healthy body. Many studies have been conducted looking at the number of babies with overt reflux (i.e. spitting up), what age it begins, and how many times it happens per day. The results are extremely variable, with one study showing overt reflux affecting 20% of babies, another showing it affected 90% of babies, and many others in between.

In most studies reflux begins early in life, with high levels from 1–5 months, after which it begins to tail off. Most studies show reflux decreasing significantly after six months (which incidentally is when most babies begin to sit upright). Vomiting may happen occasionally, once a day, or even six or more times a day.

What about colour and consistency?

Parents are often concerned about the colour of the reflux or the fact that it looks curdled. The colour and consistency of normal reflux will depend on a few factors. First it's important to realise that not all milk is actually white. If you are breastfeeding, the colour of milk can be quite variable. It can look pale and watery, it can be slightly blue, or even slightly green. It can be thick and fatty and more yellow in colour. The colour of breastmilk can vary due to diet, frequency of feeds, how full the breast was, whether baby fed at the breast or the milk was hand-expressed or pumped (these factors can affect the fat content of milk). In the early days there can even be a little blood in the milk. This may be due to trauma to the nipple due to early breastfeeding difficulties, or it sometimes just happens in the early days of feeding as milk starts to flow in the ducts (this is known as 'rusty pipe syndrome'). This can cause milk to look a little pink, orange brown or rust-coloured. Infant formula milks, in contrast, are obviously a more consistent colour and do not change from feed to feed.

Clearly the colour of milk that goes in will affect the colour of any reflux coming out. It can be very frightening to see variations of colour in refluxed milk, particularly if it looks pink. Blood in vomit should be checked out with your midwife or healthcare professional, but it's important to consider whether the blood could be coming from your milk, and expressing a little will help to determine that. If there is a little blood in your breastmilk, it will not harm your baby, although you may notice a little extra spit up until it has resolved. Any bright yellow colour in reflux should be checked with a healthcare professional as it may indicate the presence of bile.

Consistency can also vary depending on when the milk is refluxed. If the reflux or posseting happens immediately after a feed, it is likely to look much like it did when it was swallowed. If it happens a little longer after a feed, or perhaps even if the baby was feeding for a very long time, it may look slightly more curdled or lumpy. This is still entirely normal and simply means that the milk was in the baby's stomach for slightly longer and digestion had started to occur.

Reflux may seem to ooze from the baby's mouth, or it may come up more forcefully, even emerging from the baby's nose as well as mouth. It may dribble down their chin and clothes, or it may come from their mouth in an arc, landing on the floor in front of them. This is all entirely within the range of normal. How a baby reacts will also vary. Some babies are entirely unfazed by spitting up. Others will cry for a minute when it happens and then settle quickly. Reflux can be unsettling for babies even when it is entirely normal. If you have ever had a fizzy drink and have felt the gas escape through your nose, or have ever vomited and felt the vomit come through your nose you will know it's not a terribly pleasant feeling. It doesn't mean that it is painful or doing any harm, but it can certainly be unsettling and babies can cry because of it. With normal physiological reflux, babies generally settle within a few minutes, even if initially upset, if soothed by a caregiver or put to the breast. Some babies will want to feed again after refluxing, and some may just want to suck but not really be interested in more milk.

The volumes of reflux can also be quite variable. Some babies spit up so much that it may look as though they have just regurgitated their whole feed, but it is important to remember that spilt liquid often looks like more volume than it actually is. I sometimes suggest that parents take a tablespoon of liquid and pour it over their top to see how wet they get, or throw it on the floor to see how much of an area it spreads over. Usually it is very reassuring to realise what a mess a small amount of liquid can make.

What is GORD?

GORD is gastro-oesophageal reflux disease (GERD in US English). GORD may be defined as the presence of troublesome symptoms associated with reflux. Examples of troublesome symptoms can include:

- Marked distress
- Apnoea
- Hoarseness
- Unexplained feeding difficulties

- Ear infections
- Lower respiratory infections (e.g. pneumonia)
- Faltering growth
- Chronic cough
- Dental erosion
- Asthma

As many of these conditions are not solely associated with GORD, the National Institute for Health & Care Excellence (NICE) in the UK suggests that investigation for GORD should only be considered if a baby has at least two of these symptoms, and recognises that there are significant issues with diagnosis based on these symptoms.

Babies with apnoea (stoppage in breathing), hoarseness, pneumonia, cough, asthma or dental erosion certainly need medical assessment. In practice I find that many babies are diagnosed with reflux not due to any of these medical issues, but rather due to symptoms of marked distress, unexplained feeding difficulties and/or faltering growth.

It is very difficult to quantify 'marked distress' to a parent or to a healthcare provider who may be assessing a baby. In many cases excessive crying is used as a marker for distress, and often the 'rule of 3s' (Wessel's criteria) is used as a guideline. The rule of 3s is defined as crying for more than three hours a day, for at least three days a week, continuing for at least three weeks, but this is certainly not consistently applied when assessing distress. Furthermore, babies don't always get a good feeding assessment, which might explain some of the feeding problems or faltering growth, and therefore the assessment leading to a diagnosis of reflux can be quite variable.

In practice a baby with GORD is an extremely unhappy baby, and often unwell. Fortunately true GORD only affects a small number of babies. A study looking at all cases of GORD in children under 12 in the UK between 2000 and 2005 found that the rate was 0.148% in children who were a year old.[3]

What causes GORD?

The definition of GORD in babies is usually based on symptoms rather than a description of a physiological problem in the body. In many ways it is much like the diagnosis of colic. It is a diagnosis given in babies where parents describe some symptoms, rather than through any kind of diagnostic test. The working paradigm is based on adult diagnoses of 'heartburn', and the theory is that excess acid in the stomach causes pain when the stomach contents are refluxed into the oesophagus. To diagnose through a medical test the acidic nature of refluxed stomach contents can be checked using a pH probe inserted into the stomach or the oesophagus. This is clearly a very invasive process and therefore is infrequently done when parents and their family doctor are querying GORD. However, studies have been conducted which have done exactly this type of test, and the results of these cast doubt on the 'acid hypothesis' as a cause of crying in large numbers of babies.[4,5,6]

Nevertheless, the prescription of medication for GORD in babies continues to work on the acid hypothesis, and rates of prescription are increasing. A paper looking at these rates published in the *Journal of Paediatrics* in 2011 found that a US healthcare database showed that from 1999–2004 there was a seven-fold increase in PPI prescriptions.[7] PPIs are proton pump inhibitors, a class of drug which suppresses the production of stomach acid. In the same time period, one particular PPI which was a liquid formulation (and therefore easier to administer to a baby) had a 16-fold increase in prescription rate. Overall 0.5% of the babies in the database received a prescription for a PPI. Prescriptions seem to have increased worldwide since this time. A New Zealand study found that in 2012 over 5% of all babies born were prescribed PPIs.[8]

In my experience, these prescriptions are often given without parents having been given full information about what the medication does and any potential side-effects. In this book I aim to provide more information so that parents can make more informed decisions for their baby.

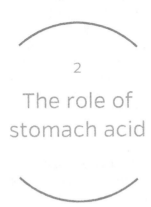

2

The role of stomach acid

Stomach acid, or gastric acid, is the digestive fluid created in the stomach. It primarily consists of hydrochloric acid (HCl), which is created by parietal cells that line the inside of the stomach wall. Other components secreted in the stomach are water, mucous (to protect the stomach lining) and pepsin (an enzyme that breaks down protein). It is estimated that an adult produces 1.5–2 litres of gastric secretions every day (0.9–1.2ml per kg of bodyweight per hour).

Studies suggest that newborns in comparison have very little secretion in the first day, with a gradual increase until the third week after birth, followed by a short decline in the third to fourth week, then rising again and reaching around the lower end of adult rates at 2–3 months.[1] By three years the amount of gastric acid produced has reached adult levels. So when considering the acid theory of reflux, it's important to realise that young infants have low levels of stomach acid in comparison to adults.

The acidity of any substance is measured on the pH scale.

Pure water is considered neutral and has a pH of 7. Substances with a pH of less than 7 are considered acidic (with 6 being weakly acidic and 2 being very acidic) and substances with a pH of more than 7 are considered alkaline (with 8 being weakly alkaline and 13 being strongly alkaline). To give some context to this, white vinegar is an acid (acetic acid) with a pH of around 2. Baking soda (sodium bicarbonate) is alkaline with a pH of around 9.

Stomach acid in digestion

The thought, smell, sight and taste of food triggers our brains to begin releasing gastric secretions in preparation for digestion. Any parent will know how their baby starts to look prepared to feed, or starts to show excitement about feeding when they hear the click of a nursing bra strap, or see a bottle approaching. The stomach begins preparing to receive milk while this is happening. When milk starts entering the stomach, the secretions increase further. A baby's tongue moves in a wave-like motion while suckling and this initiates a wave-like motion right through the whole gastro-intestinal tract, which is called peristalsis. In the stomach these wave-like contractions mix the milk and gastric secretions fully into a solution known as chyme.

Within this chyme solution, protein digestion begins. Proteins are made of long chains of small building blocks called amino acids. The long chains of amino acids fold in on themselves forming complex 3D structures. Hydrochloric acid (HCl) in the stomach acid causes these proteins to unfurl into their long chain structures. HCl also activates the pepsin enzyme which starts to break the chains apart into smaller sub-structures. This unwinding isn't just important for the digestion of proteins. It's important because many other minerals (such as calcium, iron and zinc) are bound into proteins, and can only be accessed and absorbed after the protein is unwound. The presence of stomach acid is necessary for this unwinding and subsequent digestion.

The next step in digestion is the relaxation of the sphincter muscle at the bottom of the stomach, the pyloric sphincter, which allows the chyme to pass through into the intestine. After approximately 45 minutes for a feed of breastmilk and 75 minutes for formula milk, half of the milk will have emptied from the stomach through the pyloric sphincter muscle into the intestine. Once in the intestine a large amount of bicarbonate is secreted which neutralises the acid, so the chyme becomes a neutral pH.

Stomach acid kills harmful micro-organisms

Stomach acid is also important for our immune system, and in preventing harmful micro-organisms from infecting the body.[2] Pathogenic bacterial species are destroyed within a strongly acidic environment. Even the presence of pepsin has been shown to make bacterial species more vulnerable, and it's important to remember that HCl is required in order to activate pepsin. A low-acid environment allows micro-organisms to pass through the stomach into the intestine.

We already know that young babies produce less acid than adults, so does this make them more at risk of infection due to less acid? This is where biology has put safeguards in place for the baby, in the form of milk. Breastmilk contains many anti-infective components, such as phagocytes, lymphocytes, bacteriocides and anti-viral components. Breastmilk also combines with a baby's saliva to create small amounts of hydrogen peroxide which acts as a potent anti-infective. Formula milk doesn't have any of these safeguards, which is why parents have to put their own manual safeguards in place by sterilising bottles and teats and by making up formula powder with water that has been boiled and then cooled to 70°C in order to kill pathogens that may be present in the formula.

Stomach acid and milk

Milk is an extremely good buffer of stomach acid. In other words, it neutralises acid. When a baby has a milk feed, although acid is released and mixed with the milk to form chyme, that chyme never becomes as acidic as the chyme from a typical solid non-dairy meal eaten by an adult.

A study in 2001 looked at the acid levels in the stomachs of young babies. The babies were split into three feeding groups. The first group was fed at four-hourly intervals. The second group was fed three-hourly, and the third group was fed two-hourly. To recap, a lower pH is more acidic, and a higher pH is more alkaline. A pH of 7 is neutral, like water.

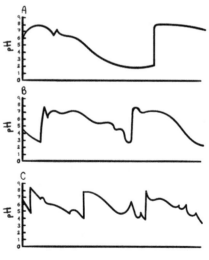

In medical terms, reflux of stomach contents which has a pH of less than 4 is considered to be acid reflux. Reflux of contents which have a pH greater than 4 is not considered to be acid reflux.

When we look at the graph we can see very clearly that each time the babies had a milk feed, the pH rose rapidly,

Figure 2: Example of pH levels in babies fed four-hourly, three-hourly and two-hourly.

neutralising the acid in the stomach. These are the large spikes upwards. With the four-hourly feeds we can see that the stomach contents have reduced to a pH of 2 before the next feed. With the three-hourly feeds the stomach contents have reduced to a pH of around 2.5 before the next feed, but with the two-hourly feeds the stomach contents have only reached a pH of 4 before the next feed. This means that the stomach contents never reached a stage where reflux would be considered to be acid reflux.

The study authors conclude that the average time it took for the gastric pH to drop to 4 was 130 minutes and that *any reflux that occurred during these periods of buffering could not be detected*.

In essence, a baby who is feeding every two hours, or more frequently, even if they are having reflux (which they likely are as it is normal), is not having acid reflux.

Young babies generally cue to feed 10–12 times a day. Some babies are placed on more rigid schedules and babies will learn to adapt to those schedules, but if held in arms and fed at the earliest cues they generally feed at least 10–12 times a day, or even more frequently. The neonatologist Nils Bergman researches mothers and babies when held in skin-to-skin contact without separation, and his research suggests that newborn babies may naturally feed every hour.[3] This makes sense when we consider the size of a small baby's stomach and the fact that breastmilk is digested easily and quickly. I understand that not everyone reading this book will be feeding their baby breastmilk, but it's important to discuss digestion in the context of breastmilk since a baby's biological digestion process has developed around the evolutionary norm of breastfeeding. Understanding how a baby drinks and digests breastmilk can help us understand how to best manage formula feeding to help babies feed most comfortably.

Feeding intervals are always counted from the start of one feed to the start of the next feed, and any parent will know that young babies often don't take a big feed in one sitting and then do the same two hours later. A baby may begin to feed, and then may need to stop to burp. They may then continue feeding. They may stop for a short rest and then start again a few minutes later. Small babies may fall asleep for 10 minutes and then wake to complete a feed. Others may need a nappy/diaper change and then drink some more. These patterns may differ slightly depending on whether your baby is feeding at the breast or feeding from a bottle, but generally feeding doesn't follow the clear patterns that these graphs suggest. More usually young babies who are fed responsively, when they cue, are topping up their stomachs with milk fairly frequently, and likely don't have much longer than 130 mins between feeds. Their stomach contents therefore wouldn't be acidic enough to constitute acid reflux. If we feed a baby on a schedule, however, or with a more rigid idea of what constitutes a feed, babies may have significantly longer than 130 mins between feeds.

The stomach acid theory of GORD

The dominant theory of GORD, which has been around for many years, is that stomach acid is refluxing into the oesophagus causing pain for the baby. Some also suggest that some babies are producing too much acid, and this is contributing to the pain. This simplistic argument might seem to make sense on the face of it, but when we look deeper it becomes more complex.

Firstly we know that babies produce lower levels of acid than adults, and secondly we know that young babies have a diet consisting solely of milk, which is a very effective buffer of stomach acid. The graph in Figure 1 shows that when a baby feeds, the stomach contents reach a neutral pH. We also know that reflux is normal and occurs in many babies, with some studies showing that it occurs in the vast majority of babies. The vast majority of babies do not have GORD, even if they are having reflux. Most babies who are spitting up or vomiting are not distressed by spitting up, and are often called 'happy spitters'. Most seem completely unconcerned. Some may grimace temporarily as it happens, perhaps not liking the taste of semi-digested milk, but are not overly distressed. What could be the difference between these babies, and the babies who are distressed by the vomiting? Why would reflux cause pain in some babies and not others?

Part of this may be explained by feeding times, since we know that babies who are fed more frequently will have a more pH neutral reflux than those who have had long gaps between feeds, but even when we consider that, it turns out that a healthy lining of the oesophagus is remarkably resistant to acid. The oesophagus is the food pipe which connects our mouth to our stomach, and the cells lining the oesophagus are specifically designed to be resistant to acid because reflux is a normal and expected process. Pepsin, for example, has the potential to break down body tissues, but research has shown that pepsin is unable to damage the oesophagus tissues at a pH of more than 3.[4] In addition to the pepsin defence, the underlying cells in the oesophagus also produce bicarbonate (which is alkaline) in order to raise the pH of stomach contents that it comes in contact with and to neutralise the acid.[5] If stomach contents have a low enough pH, and a cell is in contact with that acid long enough, these defences are compromised and acid is able to cross the border and into the cells. Even if this happens, however, the cells have a further defence mechanism that pushes that acid back out of the cells again, or takes in water to increase the pH.

With all of these mechanisms in place most people can have repeated daily episodes of reflux in which they feel no pain and there is no tissue damage. This has also been tested in studies through the Bernstein test. The Bernstein test (also known as the acid perfusion test) is a method used in labs in order to test heartburn (GORD). A nasogastric tube is passed through the nose of the patient or test subject, and down into the lower oesophagus. Hydrochloric acid is then dripped through the tube directly on to the oesophagus in order to study the reaction. Research has shown that dripping acid with a pH as low as 1.1 continuously for 30 mins in an adult person causes *no damage* to healthy oesophageal tissue. Healthy adults may be having episodes of reflux multiple times a day and be completely unaware of it, in the same way that most babies who are spitting up are unconcerned by it.

However, during the Bernstein test we see a difference between healthy adults and those who have been diagnosed with GORD. Healthy adults feel no pain and suffer no damage from the test, but those with GORD do feel pain when the oesophagus comes in contact with the acid. This seems to be because their oesophagus is already damaged and therefore the defence mechanisms are not working effectively.[6] The first line of defence for the oesophagus is maintaining a physical barrier, essentially a wall of defence along the lining of the oseophagus. This happens by the cells being tightly packed together with no gaps along the wall for the reflux to pass into. In adults with GORD it seems that this barrier wall has defects. There are gaps between the cells which allow the reflux to pass through the barrier and into the space between the cells. Once it gets in there it fires off pain receptors.

So what would cause the oesophagus lining to be damaged in the first place? Well, studies have found that people who have this 'leaky' barrier in the oseophagus have lower amounts of a protein called filaggrin.[7] Filaggrin is a sticky protein that binds the wall of the oesophagus together, a bit like mortar between bricks in a wall. Lower filaggrin has also been found in those with eczema, where there is a defect in the skin barrier, and it has been linked to hayfever, asthma and food allergy.[8,9]

Some studies have suggested a link between filaggrin gene mutations and food allergy, perhaps through sensitisation via the skin.[10] This research makes sense of what many lactation consultants like myself understand when working with babies with reflux. Normal reflux doesn't hurt babies, unless something else is already going on, like an underlying allergy. In most cases if you can identify the food allergy, remove it and allow the oesophagus tissue to heal, the reflux is no longer painful. The baby can become more like all the other happy spitters. However, there are different challenges depending on how a baby is fed. A baby who is drinking breastmilk will have lots of exposure to many anti-inflammatory and healing factors within breastmilk which will help the healing process. For these babies, finding allergens and removing them from their mother's diet can be the biggest challenge. A formula-fed baby will generally be on a cow's milk formula and if allergy is suspected, they may have to be moved to a specialised formula. Although this makes the elimination of the allergen easier, the baby is not exposed to the anti-inflammatory components of breastmilk, and amino acid formula can have its own issues, with recent concerns over mineral uptake from some amino acid formula products.[11]

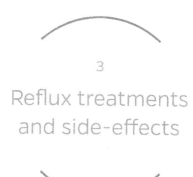

3

Reflux treatments
and side-effects

In Chapter 1 we looked at the definitions of reflux, the difference between reflux and GORD, and the fact that simple reflux is considered normal and natural in babies under the age of one. Normal reflux therefore doesn't actually require any treatment and generally resolves with time. Reflux is often confused with GORD, however, and there are many cases of babies with normal simple reflux who are being treated with drugs intended for babies with GORD. There are also many babies who are having feeding issues completely unconnected to GORD who are being treated for GORD because the feeding issues are not understood. We will look in more detail at feeding and baby care issues which can be confused with GORD in chapters 4 and 5.

There are currently three main approaches to treating reflux and GORD:

- Thickening feeds
- Alginate therapy
- Acid suppression

In this chapter I want to look at each of these approaches and explore whether they work, how they work, the side-effects, and any feeding issues to be considered.

Thickening feeds

Thickening feeds involves adding some kind of thickening agent to milk before offering it to the baby. The theory is that the thicker, heavier milk will remain in the stomach and be less likely to rise back up through the oesophagus. Thickening agents are commonly made from carob bean (also known as locust bean), rice cereal, corn starch, maize starch, xanthan gum or pectin. Preparations can be bought or prescribed in a powder which a caregiver adds to milk, and some formula milk manufacturers have created milk products with the thickener already added. A very common brand of thickener is Carobel.

Does thickening work?

That depends on the way that you look at the studies. There is no good quality evidence that shows that thickening feeds is effective in reducing reflux.[1] There are a number of studies which show that there is a reduction in the *amount* of reflux, but these studies have been graded as low to moderate quality. In fact a 2004 Cochrane Review (which reviews all available studies on a topic) concluded:

'There is no evidence from randomised controlled trials to support or refute the efficacy of feed thickeners in newborn infants with GOR... we cannot recommend using thickening agents for management of GOR in newborn infants.' [2]

Some anti-reflux milk formulas state that they reduce reflux by slowing gastric emptying due to the ratio of whey to casein milk proteins in the formula, but this claim remains controversial. Research from 2002 found that, '*Although thickened formulas do not appear to reduce measurable reflux, they may reduce vomiting.*'[3,4] In other words, the reflux changed from vomiting to 'silent reflux', where the stomach contents still left the stomach but didn't get as far as being spat out of the mouth. This might help reduce mess and laundry, but if acid is the problem issue for any particular baby (i.e. we are dealing with GORD rather than normal reflux) and this is the cause of unsettled behaviour, then simply reducing the vomit is not going to help as the reflux is still happening.

Since the studies are not conclusive, you may be tempted to try thickening milk just to see if it reduces spitting up in your baby. So the next thing we have to consider before trying any intervention is whether it does any harm.

Are there any risks to thickeners?

Firstly let's think about how thickening affects the feeding process. Thickening agents are simply not suitable for breastfeeding babies who feed either exclusively or primarily at the breast. Thickeners clearly can't be added to milk in the breasts, and therefore the only way to add them to breastmilk is to express the milk and then feed it via bottle. This disrupts breastfeeding, risks early weaning, and means that a bottle needs to be introduced (which may be contrary to the wishes of the family). It also creates twice as much effort for the caregiver since it involves both expressing (breastfeeding) and bottle-feeding, with all the associated effort of washing and sterilising bottles.

Once in the milk, thickeners change the flow, texture and taste of milk, which babies may dislike. The slower flow can also significantly increase the time taken for a feed. In fact, slowing a feed is often a good thing when it comes to reflux – but there are lots of ways to slow a feed down without using thickeners.

Secondly, let's consider whether there are any digestive side-effects to adding thickeners. Studies suggest that adding fibre (carob gum or guar gum) to milk may lower the available calcium, iron and zinc during digestion.[5] Many parents also find that thickening can be a cause of constipation in their baby. There is also a concern around preparation of thickened milk formula. Current safe formula preparation guidelines are that milk should be made up with water which has been boiled and then cooled to 70°C. The reason for this specific method is because milk powder is not sterile, and nor is water. Boiling water and then cooling it to 70°C before adding it to the milk powder is effective in killing bacteria which may be present in the water and the powder. Manufacturer guidelines for thickened formula suggest making the formula with either cold or hand warm water, as using water at 70°C may cause the thickened formula to become lumpy. This leaves the baby at higher risk of bacterial infection.

One other consideration which hasn't been looked at in studies is the fact that the use of thickeners is the addition of a foodstuff other than milk into the baby's diet, usually before the recommended weaning age.

Risks and benefits

When considering any medication for a baby we have to weigh up the potential benefits against the potential negative effects. If your baby has GORD and therefore is exhibiting marked distress when spitting up or is crying for much of the day even when in arms or at the breast, and if any feeding issues have been thoroughly assessed and resolved, then these effects on digestion may be outweighed by the benefits of a solution which is effective at reducing reflux. The evidence profile on thickeners, however, does not give us great confidence of efficacy.

If your baby is spitting up a lot but is not showing any marked distress, or settles relatively easily, then treatment should be considered more carefully.

Alginate therapy

Alginate therapy usually involves giving the baby a formulation of sodium alginate which is mixed into some milk. For a breastfed baby it is usually added into a little expressed breastmilk and given before a breastfeed, or added into the bottle of milk for a bottle-fed baby. The best known brand name for this kind of therapy is Gaviscon. The theory behind this therapy is that once the alginate product comes in contact with the stomach contents it forms a thick, gel-like solution. It also creates CO_2 (carbon dioxide) in the stomach, which then pushes the alginate gel to the top of the stomach where it acts like a raft floating on the top and prevents reflux from entering the oesophagus.[6]

Do alginates work?

Again, the evidence is not of good quality. There are studies which have shown a reduction in reflux when using alginate, but those studies have been assessed as being of low or moderate quality.[1]

Are there any risks to alginates?

As with thickeners, there may be unintended side-effects of alginate therapy. It may seem that simply creating a 'raft' wouldn't have much effect, but research does suggest a couple of potential issues.

Alginate may suppress the digestion of fats in milk. One small study of alginate therapy in adults suggested that the thick alginate gel may trap fats and fatty acids. This then reduced the amount of bile secreted to break down fats. This study also found a change (although it was not statistically significant) in the absorption of iron and manganese.[7]

A second and potentially larger concern illustrated in research is the effect on appetite. A search of research on alginate therapy brings up a wealth of studies using alginate as a therapy for obesity. Some of these studies show greater weight loss in adult obese patients when on alginate therapy, with some finding that alginate decreases appetite.[8,9,10] Studies suggest that the thick gel formed in the stomach by the alginate distends the stomach, causing the stomach to feel fuller, which prompts the individual to reduce intake.[11] This might be a desirable outcome in an obese adult, but is less so in a very young baby who needs to double their birthweight in the first six months. In practice this worries me in babies who may already not be gaining well.

Many babies who are diagnosed with silent reflux have low weight gain, are unsettled, and have fussy feeding behaviours, such as back arching while feeding. These behaviours may be misdiagnosed as being due to pain from acid and so therapy for reflux is begun. In fact, these behaviours may be due to other feeding problems. Babies who are not feeding well and are not getting enough milk because of these feeding issues can be unsettled due to hunger and frustration. Babies who are finding it hard to get flow from the bottle due to the teat shape/texture or flow rate may arch when feeding. Babies feeding at the breast often arch their back when the flow slows down as the breast empties. This arching can be a communication from the baby that they want to switch sides. For babies such as these, the solution to the unsettled crying and arching is to increase milk intake, and help them to manage that milk intake rather than to suppress appetite. Suppressing appetite may lower weight gain further and lead to further medication. Chapter 5 looks at symptoms commonly diagnosed as reflux and whether they could be due to other issues.

Risks and benefits

When considering alginate therapy we again have to weigh up the potential benefits against the potential negative effects. If your baby has GORD and therefore is exhibiting marked distress when spitting up or is crying for much of the day even when in arms and being responded to, and if all feeding issues have been thoroughly assessed and resolved, and your baby is gaining weight well, then these effects on digestion and appetite may be outweighed by the benefits of a solution which is effective. Just as with thickeners, however, the evidence profile for alginate does not give us good confidence in efficacy for any individual baby.

If your baby is spitting up a lot but is not showing any marked distress, or is already having issues with weight gain, then treatment should be considered more carefully.

Is reducing spit-up a good thing?

Both thickeners and alginate formulations are designed to stop vomiting, but is that in itself a desirable outcome? In Chapter 1 we discussed how TLOSRs act as an overflow mechanism to allow excess milk or gas to escape. Young babies have a strong physiological need to suckle, and this need isn't always about hunger. Suckling helps to stabilise and calm babies. The rhythmic motion of suckling helps to regulate their heart rate and their breathing, among other things, and newborns usually choose to spend large amounts of their time suckling. This suckling often leads to large milk intake and this can easily create an overfull stomach. A breastfeeding baby, for example, may feed, become full and fall asleep at the breast while still latched on. Babies continue to suckle while asleep and while comforting and soothing at the breast during their sleep, they may trigger another milk ejection, and suddenly take in another large volume of milk, overfilling the stomach. They may later spit up, feed again and go back to sleep. This is normal, natural and nothing to be concerned about. Newborns are still learning to breastfeed, and later will learn different ways of suckling at the breast depending on whether they just want comfort or are hungry. In the newborn stage it is best that all suckling is done at the breast and it is great for building milk supply.

'I know now that a lot of his symptoms were normal for a baby of his age and most of the time he is a 'happy sicker', i.e. he isn't distressed by being sick, so it's fine and we don't need to worry. I wish I'd had this information earlier as I would have been less anxious.' Emma

A bottle-feeding baby has a slightly different dynamic when feeding. Milk doesn't flow at a constant rate from the breast. There are periods of fast flow (where oxytocin triggers a milk ejection) and periods of slow and low volume flow between those milk ejections. With a bottle the flow rate depends primarily on the caregiver and how the bottle is being offered. If the bottle is tipped up and the baby is sucking, milk will flow at a pretty constant rate. A baby may fill their stomach but have a need to continue sucking for some other physiological regulation, or may want to suck in order to calm their nervous system so they can drift off to sleep. As the baby continues sucking from the tipped bottle, milk continues to flow and so the baby may take in a larger volume than they wanted and the stomach may become overfull. Again, the baby may then spit up the overflow and then want to suck again. In these cases spitting up is helpful and makes the baby feel more comfortable. Preventing that spit up from happening can leave the baby with a feeling of bloating and discomfort, and I have had a number of clients who came to see me after finding that their baby seemed more uncomfortable when they were on therapy to prevent spitting up.

Finally, spitting up breastmilk could even be protective. Breastmilk is full of anti-inflammatory, anti-infective components. When a baby drinks breastmilk, these components bathe the lining of the oesophagus. When a baby refluxes, the oesophagus is again bathed in these protective factors. Canadian paediatrician and breastfeeding specialist Jack Newman says:

'Breastmilk is full of immune factors (not just antibodies, but dozens of factors that interact with each other) that protect the baby from invasion by bacteria and other microorganisms (fungi, viruses, etc.) by forming a protective layer on his mucous membranes (the linings of the gut, respiratory tract and other areas). This protective layer prevents micro-organisms from invading the body through these mucous membranes. A baby who spits up gets extra protection, first when the milk goes down to the stomach, and again when he spits it up.'

Dr Jack Newman's Guide to Breastfeeding (updated edition), Jack Newman and Teresa Pitman, 2014, p124.[12]

Acid suppression

Acid suppression therapy reduces the amount of acid produced by the stomach, in order to reduce the acid content of reflux, and therefore limit any damage done by that reflux. Before we look at how acid is suppressed it's helpful to have an overview of how acid is produced in the stomach from the parietal cells which line the stomach.

1. Gastrin (a hormone) is released when food enters the stomach

2. Gastrin causes specialised stomach cells to produce histamine

3. Histamine binds to receptors on parietal cells in the stomach lining. Binding causes parietal cells to pump out hydrogen ions. This is called the proton pump

4. Hydrogen pumped out by the parietal cells combines with chloride to form hydrochloric acid (Stomach acid)

Figure 3: Production of stomach acid

There are two separate types of medication which are used to suppress acid: proton pump inhibitors (PPIs) and H2 blockers (histamine 2 blockers). Each of these has a different method of reducing acid suppression due to the particular point at which they act in the production of acid.

- *Proton pump inhibitors*
  These medications are the most potent inhibitors of acid available. PPIs intervene at stage three of the flow chart above. They stop the parietal cells from pumping out hydrogen ions and therefore prevent the creation of HCl. With less acid volume created, the stomach contents become less acidic. Examples of PPIs used in babies include omeprazole, lansoprazole and esomeprazole. Studies do back up the biology and show that babies who are treated with PPIs have a higher pH in their stomach during treatment, spending longer times at a pH above 4 (less acidic), but studies do also raise concerns about dosing in babies compared to adults.

- *H2 blockers*
  H2 blockers are so named because they block the action of histamine in the acid creation flow. Think of step three as a lock and key mechanism. The parietal cells contain the lock and histamine acts as the key. Once the key is in the lock it switches on the proton pump. H2 blockers are drugs which also fit into the parietal cell lock mechanism. The H2 blockers attach to the lock mechanism and prevent histamine from attaching to the lock. Thus the flow is blocked at this point and the proton pump is never activated.

Both forms of acid suppression have a very specific biological action and studies show that both methods do reduce the creation of acid in the stomach and increase the pH of the stomach contents. If acid was the cause of reflux symptoms, this might seem to be the perfect solution, but unfortunately it is not that simple.

Does acid suppression work?

A review of five trials which compared PPIs against a placebo (i.e. a substance that we know will have no effect) found that PPIs were not effective in reducing GORD symptoms in babies.[13] A study looking at lansoprazole use in infants found no difference between lansoprazole and placebo in reducing feeding-related crying.[14] Another double-blinded, placebo-controlled trial looking specifically at omeprazole found that although the omeprazole increased the stomach pH and reduced the number of reflux episodes, it didn't reduce the amount of crying or fussiness.[15] This would suggest that acid exposure wasn't the cause of the crying even though the babies had been diagnosed with GORD.

The efficacy of PPIs in reducing reflux symptoms in babies is therefore not conclusive.

Are there any risks to acid suppression?

Next let's look at the side-effects. We can start with the side-effects listed in the patient insert leaflet. The common PPIs used where I work are omeprazole, esomeprazole and lansoprazole. The patient leaflets list headache, stomach pain, wind, constipation, diarrhea, nausea and vomiting as *common* side-effects for these drugs.[16,17,18] It's notable that generally the drug is often prescribed to reduce vomiting, yet a common side-effect is vomiting! Also notable is that the patient insert leaflet for these drugs states that they should not be used in infants. When we use them in infants it is an off-licence use.

Many studies have expressed concern about the use of acid suppression in babies, for multiple reasons. Dosing has been raised as a concern by some. Ward and Kearns noted in 2013, for example, that babies receive much higher doses of PPI drugs than adults. They stated:

'The volume of gastric acid that is released after stimulation relates to the parietal cell mass and does not reach adult levels until 5–6 months after birth. Although it would seem logical that a smaller parietal cell mass would require smaller doses of a PPI for inhibition, that is not the case, or at least that is not current practice. When the current neonatal and infant doses of PPI are compared with the capacity for acid secretion in milliEquivalents, these doses are 7-fold to 9-fold higher than the doses that are effective for treatment of adults.' [19]

The authors conclude that more research is needed to look at dosages in babies.

However, it's not only dosages that are concerning, but also the consequences of reducing stomach acid. Stomach acid is vital for correcting metabolism, breaking down proteins, and for the availability of various vitamins and minerals to the body. Research suggests that PPIs may lower levels of vitamin B12, vitamin C, iron and magnesium in the body.[20] Indeed, the patient leaflet for lansoprazole states that the medication may lead to a reduced absorption of B12.

Several studies have found that those taking acid-suppressing drugs have higher rates of respiratory infections, fractures, pneumonia and gastro-intestinal infections. Most of the studies have been done on adults or older children, but a recent study looking at fractures in children seems to back up the concern. This study looked at almost 875,000 children born between 2001 and 2013 and found that children who received PPIs in the first six months of life had a 22% increased risk of a bone fracture in the next six years.[21] If the baby was taking both PPIs and an H2 blocker the increased risk of a fracture was 31%. The researchers also found a dose-dependent link. Babies who took PPIs for less than a month had a 19% greater risk of a bone break, while babies taking them for longer than five months were at a 42% increased risk. I find this extremely worrying. My experience of working with babies is that babies are often prescribed acid suppressants in the first few weeks of life and continue on the treatment until they are on solids at around six months. I have not met any parents who were informed of these risks when the drug was prescribed.

Dr Malchodi, who conducted the study, told the attendees of the 2017 Pediatric Academic Societies Meeting:

'our study adds to a growing body of evidence suggesting [acid-reducing] medications are not safe for children, especially very young children... they should only be prescribed to treat confirmed serious cases of more severe, symptomatic, gastroesophageal reflux disease (GERD), and for the shortest length of time needed.'

There has also been a study done in babies which backs up the link with increased infections. The study comparing lansoprazole and placebo mentioned above found that although treating with the PPI didn't reduce the symptoms attributed to GORD, there was a significant increase in infections in the babies treated, particularly lower respiratory infections.

If this wasn't concerning enough, there is also research to suggest that acid suppression could play a role in the development of food allergy. When we are allergic to any particular food, it is most often the proteins which cause the allergic reaction. This is why an allergy to dairy products is usually referred to as CMPA (cow's milk protein allergy). The breakdown of proteins is necessary to lessen the allergic potential of any food, and stomach acid is essential for that. A 2013 study looking at almost 5,000 children diagnosed with GORD found that those who were treated with acid suppressants were 68% more likely to be diagnosed with a food allergy than those who weren't.[22] Food allergy may be more likely in children diagnosed with GORD anyway, and may cause symptoms of GORD (more on this later), but this study concluded it was the acid suppression which raised the risk of food allergy diagnosis. The study stated that it highlighted *'the importance of the judicious use of these medications, especially in the pediatric population'*.

When you look at these side-effects and implications, together with the number of children who are being treated with acid suppressants, it paints a fairly concerning picture.

Risks and benefits

As with the previous therapies, when considering treating a baby with acid suppressants we need to weigh up whether the benefit conferred by the treatment outweighs the side-effects that we have mentioned. Again this will depend on whether your baby has normal reflux or GORD. If your baby isn't exhibiting distressed behaviour when spitting up then it's important to realise that your baby likely just has normal reflux, which requires no treatment at all.

If your baby is clearly distressed by spitting up, or by reflux which isn't being vomited, then you may feel some of these side-effects are worth it if the treatment is used for a short time. However, the evidence for PPIs being effective in reducing crying and distressed behaviour is inconclusive. When considering reduction of stomach acid, it's important to remember that acid shouldn't hurt a healthy oesophagus (see Chapter 2). It does cause instant pain to an oesophagus which is already damaged due to something like food allergy, however, so allergy should also be investigated. Chapter 5 deals with allergy and identifying possible allergy in your baby. In the case of allergy, removing the allergen from the diet can turn GORD back into normal reflux and mean that acid suppressants can be avoided or discontinued.

Weaning off acid suppressants

A final word on stopping acid suppressants. Whereas thickeners and alginate treatment can just be stopped at any time, acid suppressants need to be tapered off to prevent a rebound effect (i.e. secretion of excess acid). Eating, or the expectation of food, starts the process of acid secretion in the stomach, and the flow chart in Figure 1 shows that the start of this process is secretion of gastrin. If the stomach is prevented from creating HCl by an acid suppressant, the stomach produces more and more gastrin in an attempt to create HCl to allow digestion to work correctly. Gastrin levels therefore increase in the blood. If you suddenly remove the acid suppression treatment, the increased gastrin levels result in much larger production of HCl than normal, so the patient/baby suddenly does have too much acid. This can take 1–2 weeks to normalise.

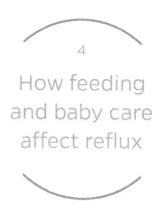

4

How feeding
and baby care
affect reflux

Simple, uncomplicated reflux is normal and physiological in young babies, but it is certainly affected by the way they are fed. How we feed our babies, what we feed them, how often we feed them, and how we interact with them all play a role in the reflux symptoms or GORD symptoms that we see.

Parenting differs across the world, and the way that we parent in the Western world has changed enormously since industrialisation. Unfortunately this means that in order to fit our babies into an industrialised society, we have lost touch with many normal infant behaviours and their communications and needs. This leads to us misinterpreting many behaviours and signals. Learning to tap into these again can help us to understand many of the behaviours often attributed to GORD.

Frequency and volume of feeds
This is the first area where biological norms often run into

conflict with cultural expectations of what is a normal feeding frequency, or in other words the first area where our baby's expectations run into conflict with what society tells us babies *should* do. The WHO and UNICEF Baby Friendly Hospital Initiative tell new mothers that babies need to feed 8–12 times a day. Quite often eight times a day is emphasised, and there is a very good reason for that. It's because eight is the bare minimum number of times that we can expect a newborn to feed and still gain weight acceptably. It is the rock bottom floor of feeding, and it is this floor that society has seemingly adopted as the standard. So we expect babies to feed three-hourly. Rather than seeing it as a minimum, Western societies, so driven by targets, have adopted the three-hourly feed as a goal, and that is the message that new parents get. Within a very short time there is an expectation that this will increase to more of a four-hourly schedule. The biological norm is, in fact, very far removed from this.

The Swedish neonatologist Nils Bergman is world renowned for his research into the importance of skin-to-skin after birth and instinctive infant feeding behaviours. His research suggests that a physiologically normal feeding frequency is probably more likely to be one-hourly![1] A newborn baby's stomach holds on average around 20ml. A 3kg baby will need around 480ml a day (after the colostrum phase). A baby feeding every three hours will need to drink 60ml at each feed to meet this amount over 24 hours. A baby feeding every hour, in contrast, will need to drink 20ml at each feed, which is – not coincidentally – the comfortable capacity of the stomach. It also takes about 45 minutes for the stomach to empty of breastmilk, so it makes sense that the baby would be ready to feed again shortly after this. The emptying time is longer for formula, and you may be using formula for your baby, but when talking about physiology it helps to think about how the stomach and metabolism developed alongside breastmilk and the digestion of breastmilk. We also find that a baby's blood sugar dips around 90 mins after a feed. This metabolic design also fits neatly with frequent feeding to prevent that blood sugar dip.

What happens if we try to put 60ml into a stomach which only comfortably holds 20ml? It overflows and we get reflux. The stomach will stretch to a certain degree, but there is a comfort level to this. Think about a time that you have overeaten, and the discomfort that you have felt. I imagine that expanding the stomach to three times its usual capacity would feel quite unpleasant, and might result in quite a bit of overflow.

The size of the stomach does increase with age, and we can see that babies increase the amount that they take per feed as the weeks pass. The amounts can be different for babies feeding at the breast and babies feeding with a bottle. When drinking at the breast we might consider 4oz (120ml) to be a full feed for a six-week-old baby, whereas the same baby when bottle-fed might drink 6oz (180ml). That difference is often dependent on how we give the bottle of milk.

From around six weeks until six months a breastfed baby will drink, on average, around 28oz of milk a day and each feed might be around 3–5oz (90–150ml). After six months the amount decreases as the baby begins on solids and the dependence on milk gradually reduces. This often surprises people who are used to seeing formula feeding, where a baby increases from 4oz milk feeds, to 6oz milk feeds, and possibly up to 8oz milk feeds. Larger volumes mean less frequent feeds, so we can often get very different feeding patterns for breastfeeding and formula-feeding babies. If we take 28oz as the average figure, a baby who is feeding every 90 minutes will need to drink 2–3oz at each feed. A baby feeding every three hours will need to take 3–4oz at each feed. A baby feeding every four hours will need to take 4–5oz at each feed. A baby's feeding isn't as regular as this of course – often babies will cluster some feeds closer together and usually have one period during 24 hours where they take a longer sleep. That may or may not be at night time, but it does mean that feeds don't have defined times and amounts.

The cultural push in the Western world to increase the length of time between a baby's feeds is strange. It seems to be based around the idea that feeding is inconvenient, and a desire to make it easy and less time-consuming for the caregiver rather than looking at the best options for the baby. In fact when feeding time is looked at with a cold analytical eye, it is frequent feeding which is less time-consuming. If we look again at a 3kg newborn breastfeeding at the breast, that baby will elicit a milk ejection reflex within 1–2 minutes of beginning suckling. Often it is within a few seconds. That milk ejection has around 30ml on average and takes about 1–2 minutes to deliver.[2] The newborn then often falls asleep at the breast. The total feeding time is around 3–5 minutes. The baby will usually continue suckling while sleeping, but the active feeding is over. In contrast a baby who is feeding three-hourly will need to drink 60ml. Feeding this amount by bottle might take around 15 minutes, followed by five minutes of burping and reflux due to discomfort from the stretching of the stomach, so a total of 20 minutes. Nils Bergman points out that hourly feeding takes 72 minutes in total (3 x 24) whereas the three-hourly feeding takes 160 mins (8 x 20).

Recently, when discussing frequent feeding with a family, a mother asked, 'How long do you just keep feeding frequently on demand like that? Is it forever?' I thought for a moment, and suggested that actually it was forever, and that when she felt hungry or thirsty she probably walked to the kitchen and got a snack or a glass of water, and was feeding herself on demand. We often don't consider how often we are 'feeding' as adults. If you count each glass of water, each cup of tea/coffee and each small bite we put in our mouths, we feed pretty frequently during the day too. As adults we are often advised to have eight glasses of water a day for example, which is often a drink every couple of hours, without considering the food. As adults we eat and drink this frequently when we are trying to maintain our weight. Babies are trying to double their birth weight in the first six months, so small frequent meals make sense, as does the idea that if you overfill a container it overflows.

Takeaway

Reflux is more likely with larger, more infrequent feeds. Reflux is less likely with smaller, frequent feeds.

Positioning and stress

Studies on reflux often find that reflux significantly improves after six months. There are very good reasons for this. At six months babies usually begin sitting up, and to do that their core muscles have to be well developed. Their core needs to be able to hold the body upright, and an upright body is less likely to experience vomiting than a horizontal body that may have milk sloshing around the oesophagheal sphincter. A very young baby does not have this muscle control and relies on parents and caregivers to provide that upright positioning, by being carried upright against their body. Where traditionally babies were carried in makeshift slings, in Western society we have more of a 'container culture' for babies. The 'container baby' is a relatively new term arising in healthcare and childcare settings, which really describes babies who spend a lot of time in enclosed spaces, such as car seats, bouncy or vibrating chairs, swings, nests, prams, strollers, cribs and baskets. Each of these 'containers' generally keeps babies in a horizontal or reclined position rather than upright, and this has implications for development.[3] Horizontal time is needed – but it's needed in the form of tummy time, rather than time on the back, and the amount of tummy time a baby gets affects whether that baby has the core muscle development and coordination skills to sit upright at six months. This development and skill development will affect the level of reflux a baby has.

Reflux is often diagnosed when a baby doesn't like to be laid down on their back – but in fact it is completely normal for many young babies not to like being laid on their back. Babies have higher arousal levels when they are on their back than when lying on their stomach.[4] In layman's terms that means that they are less relaxed/more stressed. Newborns are more likely to show the startle reflex (Moro reflex) when lying on their back than on their stomach. Likewise we also see that preterm babies have less crying and fewer stress responses when lying on their stomach. Lying on the back may be a mild stressor for a baby, and indeed some researchers suggest it is the state of mild stress which makes it successful in reducing rates of SIDS.[5] It prevents babies getting so relaxed that they fall into a deep sleep from which a vulnerable, at-risk baby may not rouse.

Being in a state of mild stress isn't good for us all the time though, so it is important for babies to also spend time on their stomachs. When the Back to Sleep campaign was launched, it was recognised that there needed to be a joint focus on tummy time – Back to Sleep, Tummy to Play. Tummy time is vital for babies to allow correct physical development, and unfortunately our container culture limits the amount of time that our babies spend on their tummies. Studies show that physical development is now delayed compared to the time before the Back to Sleep campaign was introduced. A 2005 study looking at sleep positioning and motor development found that at six months only 22% of the babies could sit without arm support, when 50% would be expected. The authors stated:

'Typically developing infants who were sleep-positioned in supine had delayed motor development by age 6 months, and this was significantly associated with limited exposure to awake prone positioning.'[6]

These types of delays are seen as early as two months, with delayed ability to lift the head well, and when a baby can roll over and even pull to stand or to walk.[7] Back to Sleep has been clearly shown to reduce SIDS, so none of these studies are recommending that babies are no longer put on their backs to sleep; rather, they are illustrating the importance of babies being placed on their front during awake time. This feeds into reflux because of the overall core strength being developed, which helps reduce vomiting through positioning. More tummy time is helpful. In fact the research suggests that a baby should be getting around 90 minutes of tummy time each day. Many of our babies diagnosed with reflux are not getting that time.[8]

Lying on the stomach may also reduce episodes of reflux. Parents are often reluctant to put babies on their stomach in the fear that pressure on the stomach will cause reflux, but the research doesn't show this to be the case. A 2007 study looking at preterm infants found fewer episodes of reflux if the babies were on their fronts or lying on their left side.[9]

A good way to combine upright positioning with tummy

contact in a newborn is carrying the baby against the body (e.g. in arms or a sling using the UK Sling Consortium's TICKS guidelines – see babyslingsafety.co.uk), or allowing the baby to sleep prone on the caregiver's chest (while the caregiver is awake and alert). This may have four effects which help with reflux.

1. It provides upright positioning which may reduce episodes of reflux.
2. It provides some tummy time which adds to ongoing physical development.
3. It allows the caregiver to pick up the earliest possible feeding cues, which then allows for small frequent feeds.
4. It reduces stress for the baby – and often also for the caregiver. The baby will still need horizontal tummy time for optimal development, but carrying/baby wearing is a good start.

Why would reducing stress make a difference? A 2010 study of adult volunteers found more TLOSRs and reflux episodes at times when cardiac vagal tone was low.[10] Cardiac vagal tone is often used as a sign of a stress response. In other words, stress may be linked to more frequent reflux. A 2001 study looking at patients who experienced sensitivity to reflux compared to those who didn't found that sensitive patients had lower vagal tone (i.e. were more stressed).[11]

Nils Bergman, who intensively studies newborn babies, says that babies feel stressed when they are separated from their mother or caregiver. He states that when not being held 'the newborn brain feels unsafe, it perceives danger and threat to life, and its basic needs are not provided.'[12]

Holding a baby more can make a big difference to babies

who are unsettled as well as potentially reducing reflux episodes. In fact research tells us that in a culture (the !Kung San tribe) where babies are carried in slings for most of the day, feed very frequently and are responded to swiftly, the babies cry for about 10 minutes a day.[13] This is in stark contrast to UK babies who cry much more. Studies show that UK babies are carried much less, are fed less frequently and there tends to be more of a delay in responding to babies when they signal a need.[14]

Takeaway

Babies have evolved to be upright against a body rather than in containers, or lying on their back for much of the day. Upright positioning reduces reflux. When against a body, babies are more relaxed. Stressed bodies have more reflux than relaxed bodies. Babies cry significantly less if carried for most of the day and responded to promptly.

Burping

Burping babies can be a very cultural idea. Where I live, burping is seen as an essential thing to do after feeding a baby. Babies are frequently woken after having drifted peacefully to sleep during a feed, in order to burp them. Often this isn't intentional, but sitting the baby up after the feed and the process of winding wakes them. Not surprisingly, the baby often wants to feed again, since the rhythmic suckling relaxes and calms them and helps them to drift back to sleep. The second feed, however, may well lead to overfilling the tummy, and a little bit of reflux.

Sometimes parents don't want to feed the baby again, as they feel that the feed is now over, and this causes the baby to cry. The crying is then often immediately blamed on wind, and not having been adequately burped. Burping isn't something which is practised the world over, and there isn't really research to back it up as helpful or needed. In fact it's possible that for some babies it is positively unhelpful. A study published in *Child: Care, Health and Development* in 2015 looking at 71 mother/baby pairs found that babies who were burped spat up over twice as often as babies who weren't burped.[15] They also found no difference in crying time. It's a small study but an interesting one, particularly when I find that many parents worry about not being able to get their baby's 'wind up' when in fact the baby simply doesn't need to burp right then. The baby just doesn't have wind.

Babies generally let us know if they need to burp. When feeding they may grimace, squirm or pop on and off the breast or the bottle, and often at this point if we set them upright and give them a gentle back rub, or gently rock them back and forth it is enough to help relieve that wind. If sleeping on your chest, shoulder, or against your body in a sling they often squirm and give themselves a gentle tummy massage and work the air out themselves. Again a gentle rub or change in position can help them at this stage, but I question whether a ritual of burping after every feed is necessary.

Takeaway

Babies may not need to be winded or burped after every feed. If they fall asleep during the feed, then allowing them to sleep on their tummy over your shoulder may help to get any air out without active 'burping'.

Sleeping environment

Sleep, the general night-time sleep environment and its effect on reflux can look very confusing at first glance. I have known many parents who say that their baby is very unsettled during the day (often having been diagnosed with silent reflux) yet they feed and sleep well beside mum at night. Others report that their baby is settled during the day, but waking frequently at night or vomiting frequently at night when laid down. An incredible array of props and tools are marketed to aid with reflux and sleep. These can range from wedge pillows for babies, props to raise one side of the cot and even vibrating cushions where a baby sleeps on their front.

So what does the research tell us about normal infant sleep, and reflux? In 1990 the *Journal of Paediatrics* published an article looking at elevating the head above the stomach in an effort to reduce reflux. 90% of the babies in the study had been categorised as having an abnormal degree of reflux and in these babies there was no significant difference in reflux between those that had their heads raised and those that were lying flat.[16] This was backed up by a 1997 study looking at sleep postioning and reflux which concluded that head elevation did not have any significant effect and therefore may not be of any clinical value in managing reflux.[17] They did find that sleeping on the left side was effective in reducing reflux however, just as it is in adults.

At this point it's important to point out that although tummy sleep or side sleep does appear to reduce reflux, it does not meet current safe sleep guidelines. Joint recommendations from the North American Society for Paediatric Gastroenterology, Hepatology and Nutrition (NASPGHAN) and the European Society for Paediatric Gastroenterology, Hepatology and Nutrition (ESPGHAN) state that:

'Prone positioning decreases the amount of acid esophageal exposure measured by pH probe compared with that measured in the supine position. However, prone and lateral positions are associated with an increased incidence of sudden infant death syndrome

(SIDS). The risk of SIDS outweighs the benefit of prone or lateral sleep position on GER; therefore, in most infants from birth to 12 months of age, supine positioning during sleep is recommended.' [18]

There does not seem to be any good quality evidence that raising a baby's head while sleeping has a significant effect on reflux, and of course lying mostly flat with a slight elevation (as happens when using wedge cushions or elevating one side of the cot) is very different to the upright positioning of a baby being held upright against a body during the day. If you are considering left lateral sleep or tummy sleep, talk to your care provider and make an informed decision about safety, as the research on back sleeping shows clearly that it reduces the risk of SIDS.

Parents have described their fear of reflux to me, and their experience of their baby having a moment where they stopped breathing (apnoea). Newborns do have an immature respiratory centre, and this is part of what places them at increased risk of SIDS. In 1992 a study looked at 100 babies with reflux, 50 of whom had had a potentially life-threatening stoppage of breathing during their sleep. These babies were studied to see if the reflux caused these events. Over 7,000 apnoeas (stoppages of breath) were noted during the study, but in the five minutes before and after any reflux episodes there were no differences in apnoeas noted, so the researchers concluded that the reflux episodes were not related to apnoea. [19]

What is happening with the babies who seem settled all day while being held after feeds, but are extremely unsettled at night? For many babies the difference is in the physical contact. In the day they are held close as the parent has been advised to keep them upright after feeds, but at night they are laid down alone in a cot or crib. Our babies are born as very immature mammals, and evolutionary biologists say that they are best thought of as exterogestates in the early months after birth. In other words, they have not completed their gestation when they are born. They complete it outside the womb. They are designed to be held close and to be in constant or almost-constant contact with us. Being out of contact with their caregiver raises stress levels. Indeed, a baby's brainwave patterns and sleep cycles are different when sleeping with a caregiver than when sleeping alone, so babies are aware of separation even when asleep.[20] This separation could be a very short distance i.e. sleeping in a cot a short way from mum's bed.

Separation leads to a stress state in babies, increased episodes where they stop breathing, increased cortisol (a stress hormone), and less feeding (not good for a young baby who needs to double their birthweight in six months). We also know that stress increases the risk of reflux as it can loosen the LOS muscle and that can increase reflux. For the families who find that their baby is content during the day but are concerned about reflux (particularly silent reflux) at night, separation may be a factor. For those who co-sleep and find that their baby seems less bothered by reflux at night, this may be due to a nurturing, evolutionarily normal sleep environment with no separation.

Takeaway

Babies are born immature and normal body function relies on being close to an adult. Being separated and placed on their back creates a slight stress situation. This stress reduces the risk of SIDS, but increases the risk of being unsettled and of having reflux.

Milk type and composition

The type of milk a baby gets (breastmilk or formula milk) doesn't just have a potential impact on volumes and frequency of feeding. The type of milk also directly impacts the rate of reflux. Studies show that breastfed babies have significantly less refluxing time, and the reflux takes a shorter time to resolve.[21,22]

There may be many reasons for this other than feeding frequency and volume. It may be due to the fact that formula stays in the stomach much longer than breastmilk and so makes reflux more possible.[23] It may be due to the different metabolic profile of formula (different amounts and types of protein, fats, sugars) to breastmilk. It may also be due to hypersensitivity to non-human milk proteins. Cow's milk protein allergy or intolerance is a growing issue for our babies. A baby who reacts to cow's milk protein may also react to goat's milk protein, and potentially other non-human milk proteins (such as soy), so choosing a non-cow's milk formula doesn't always resolve the problem.

Food hypersensitivity is covered in more detail in Chapter 5, but it's important to say here that if you are using formula for your baby and you now would like to breastfeed due to concern about reflux, then it is possible to do so. Relactation can happen weeks or months after your baby is born, and indeed adoptive mothers can induce lactation to feed their adopted baby. It is a time-consuming process but most people who do it find it extremely rewarding. If it is something you want to get some guidance about, find an IBCLC (International Board Certified Lactation Consultant) near you, or a breastfeeding organisation such as La Leche League.

Takeaway

Formula-fed babies have more reflux than breastfed babies. Cow's milk protein allergy can also be a cause of reflux symptoms. It is possible to relactate if you wish to give your baby breastmilk.

LOS 'looseners'

In adults, research suggests that a number of hormones, chemicals and foods can decrease lower oesophageal sphincter (LOS) tone and lead to reflux, such as caffeine, alcohol, smoking, chocolate and some medications such as calcium channel blockers.

A baby who is around smoke, or someone who has been smoking, may be more likely to have reflux, and reducing or removing smoke exposure will benefit them by possibly reducing reflux episodes.

Caffeine as a culprit for excessive reflux is more applicable to a breastfed baby than one who is formula-fed. When we ingest caffeine it passes into our bloodstream and, if breastfeeding, it then passes into our milk. Higher levels of caffeine have the potential to create episodes of reflux in a baby by reducing tone of the LOS. Young babies take much longer to metabolise caffeine than adults. The half-life of caffeine in an adult (the length of time it takes for half of the caffeine to be completely metabolised) is 4.9 hours. In a newborn, however, it is around 97.5 hours![24] By around four months that has decreased to 14 hours and by six months it is actually lower than an adult. This means that for a newborn the amount of time needed to metabolise caffeine is almost 20 times longer than for an adult. This means that if a breastfeeding parent is having multiple caffeine intakes during the day it can bioaccumulate in the baby and has the potential to increase reflux episodes. This doesn't mean that you can't have caffeine when breastfeeding. A moderate amount of caffeine is unlikely to have any big effect, and caffeine is actually used in treating premature babies with breathing difficulties. If you are breastfeeding, have a baby who is refluxing excessively, have worked through feeding frequency, volume, positioning and so on and you enjoy several espressos a day, it might be worth considering if the volume of caffeine you are consuming may be contributing to your baby's symptoms.

Caffeine intake is not a common cause of infant reflux, but I can think of one mother and baby I worked with where the baby was possetting several times each hour. As we worked through the case history the mother mentioned that each time she sat down to feed her baby she had a cup of tea or coffee. With a young baby who feeds frequently that's a lot of cups! When the mother reduced her intake of caffeine the reflux instantly reduced to a normal level. A small 1997 study in adults with reflux also found that switching their normal caffeinated breakfast coffee to a decaffeinated version reduced their reflux.[25]

One of the great advantages of breastfeeding is that we can, to some degree, make modifications to milk that can be helpful by slightly altering diet where we need to, in a way that isn't possible with formula.

In her book *Breastfeeding Answers Made Simple*, Nancy Mohrbacher suggests that caffeine intake in excess of 750mg a day (approx five 5oz cups of coffee) may create caffeine stimulation in a baby.[26]

Chocolate is also thought to loosen the LOS in adults. Young babies are unlikely to be eating chocolate, and chocolate doesn't pass into breastmilk, but it does contain caffeine, so is potentially another route for caffeine intake, although the effect is probably small in most people.

Takeaway

Smoke is a big factor in reflux. In some breastfeeding babies, diet can also have an impact. Reducing smoke exposure reduces reflux.

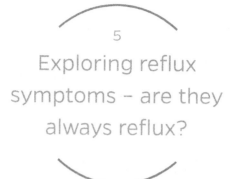

5

Exploring reflux symptoms – are they always reflux?

The range of behaviours that are often considered to be reflux symptoms is wide and varied. Behaviours which are often listed as being symptomatic of reflux on health, parenting and infant feeding websites, blogs and podcasts often include the following:

- Spitting up milk
- Feeding difficulties e.g. gagging, choking, refusing feeds
- Frequent hiccups
- Frequent coughing
- Excessive crying
- Crying during feeding
- Crying after feeding
- Arching during feeds
- Waking often at night
- Comfort feeding or frequent feeding
- Poor weight gain
- Green or yellow vomit or vomit with blood

- Recurrent pneumonia
- Projectile vomiting
- Colicky or windy
- High weight gain
- Trouble with self-settling
- Hoarse voice
- Teeth that show signs of acid erosion
- Wheeze
- Not comfortable lying on back
- Wants to be held constantly

Often a baby may be diagnosed with reflux if they exhibit two or more of these symptoms. Once the diagnosis is received the cycle of medication often begins.

When grouped together, I find that the symptoms fall into three main categories:

Feeding behaviours	<ul><li>Spitting up milk</li><li>Frequent hiccups</li><li>Crying during feeding</li><li>Crying after feeding</li><li>Arching during feeding</li><li>Comfort feeding or frequent feeding</li><li>Poor weight gain</li><li>High weight gain</li></ul>
Unsettled behaviours	<ul><li>Excessive crying</li><li>Waking often at night</li><li>Colicky or windy</li><li>Trouble with self-settling</li><li>Not comfortable lying on back</li><li>Wants to be held constantly</li></ul>

Medical issues	• Frequent coughing • Green or yellow vomit • Blood in vomit • Recurrent pneumonia • Persistent projectile vomiting • Hoarse voice • Teeth that show signs of acid erosion • Wheeze

Babies who are experiencing any of the symptoms which I have grouped as 'Medical issues' need to be seen by a doctor. These are not symptoms of normal reflux and are generally reflective of another underlying issue or medically diagnosed GORD. They fortunately tend to be uncommon.

What I want to explore in more detail are the symptoms in the first two groups, and to explain why these are not necessarily good indicators of whether a baby has GORD. The symptoms listed are very wide-ranging, so much so that it is possible to label or self-diagnose many babies with GORD who in fact are simply displaying normal baby behaviours which have been misinterpreted.

Feeding behaviours
Spitting up milk

Spitting up is clearly reflux, but as we discussed in Chapter 1, simple reflux is normal and generally doesn't require medicating. Simple reflux is generally a laundry issue (sometimes a very onerous laundry issue), but doesn't cause the baby any distress. It may happen after occasional feeds, or after every feed. It may involve a change of a bib, or a change of clothes. It may even involve a change of clothes for the caregiver.

How do we determine if reflux is causing a baby distress? Is it as simple as a baby crying when the reflux occurs? Maybe, but maybe not. A baby may be distressed by the action of the reflux, rather than it causing any pain. Consider a baby who is lying down on his back and refluxes. An older baby may be able to roll on to their side and spit out the milk. A young baby may find themselves lying with milk in their mouth or throat while they are trying to breathe. This can threaten the airway and that could be very frightening, even if it isn't painful. Distress at reflux can potentially be emotional and psychological rather than always being due to painful acid. When the baby is lifted and soothed they may calm due to having been removed from the stressful situation. Painful reflux may not resolve so quickly.

What about the baby that cries momentarily when spitting up, even if upright – are they in pain or distress from acid? Reflux may be unpleasant at times. Milk consistency may have changed, and the taste may not be pleasant when it is partially digested in the stomach. A baby may cry due to the sensation or the taste. Again, these babies generally calm quickly and easily. They may want a quick feed, just like an adult might want a glass of water after vomiting to remove the taste.

In my experience the baby who is in pain clearly lets you know that they are in pain. Parents report that the baby does not soothe easily after spitting up. There continues to be distress for some time. Adults with GORD report the pain from GORD attacks lasting for quite protracted times – maybe even 1–2 hours. The baby may show distress while being carried, when being put to the breast, through any attempts to soothe. This is very different from the baby who cries for a minute and then soothes at the breast/botttle/pacifier, or soothes in arms.

Frequent hiccups

Hiccups are a very normal occurrence in babies both in the womb and in the weeks following birth. Hiccups are caused by the diaphragm (the large muscle across the chest) spasming and forcing air up through the vocal chords, making the characteristic 'hic' sound. It is thought that they can be triggered by an overfull stomach, but this can't be the only reason, as this doesn't seem to be the reason for hiccups before birth. There is a small association between hiccups and reflux in adults, with 10% of adults with reflux complaining of hiccups, compared to 3% without reflux, but hiccups are also noted in research to be caused by over-excitement, anxiety, stress and fear, so the triggers are not all stomach related.[1] A 1980 study monitoring 20 babies found that babies hiccupped 2.5% of the time that they were monitored, and on average hiccupping lasted for eight minutes.[2] The researchers concluded that hiccups occur frequently in all young babies.

It's clear that hiccups have multiple causes. A small study has even looked at brain activity during hiccups and found that hiccups are associated with particular electrical patterns in the brain.[3] The researchers suggested that the hiccups may even have a role in brain development. There is no evidence that hiccups are an indicator of GORD in babies. They do not cause pain and may simply be part of normal nervous system development. For the vast majority of babies hiccups resolve very quickly by giving the baby a chance to feed or to suck on a pacifier. This process brings the diaphragm back into a better rhythm and stops the spasm.

Crying during feeding

This could potentially be a sign that a baby is in pain, but very often indicates a feeding difficulty instead. There are many reasons that a baby may cry during a feed which aren't due to

GORD. In order to feed well a baby needs to be able to open their mouth wide and latch well to the breast or bottle. The nipple needs to rest deep in the mouth with pressure on the palate stimulating a suckling response. The baby needs to be able to get milk from the breast or bottle and the milk needs to flow at a rate that allows the baby to easily coordinate their suck, swallow and breathe pattern. The milk needs to continue to flow until the baby is full and ready to stop feeding, and the position that the baby is in needs to be comfortable to maintain. A number of things can interfere with easy feeding and lead to crying.

Latching difficulty

Any baby who is not well attached to the breast or bottle or doesn't have the nipple/teat in the right area of the mouth, may stop suckling and begin crying. At the breast this may look like a baby latching on, taking 2–3 sucks and then coming off crying without really having started to actively feed. On a bottle with a short teat which doesn't reach far enough back you might see your baby's mouth right around the collar of the bottle. You may also see milk leaking from the mouth, and the baby may look uncomfortable or cry. Conversely you may find that a bottle teat is too long for your baby, and in this case you might find your baby gagging when feeding and then crying. If breastfeeding, you may benefit from some support around getting a deep latch. If bottle-feeding you may benefit from a different teat/bottle combination.

Slow flow

Milk which is flowing too slowly or too quickly can also lead to a baby crying when feeding. If a hungry baby is feeding but not getting enough milk, or having to work hard to get a small amount of milk, the baby may become frustrated, cry, arch away from the breast or bottle or might start chewing on the nipple. They may wave their hands around or hit the breast. These are frustrated actions of a baby asking for more milk, but the crying and particularly the arching can frequently be misinterpreted as a silent reflux symptom.

At the breast a baby may feed happily during a milk ejection, but may become frustrated, arch away from the breast and cry once the letdown/milk ejection is over. If you are unsure of when you have a milk ejection or are having trouble identifying swallowing, figuring out if the fussing is during slow flow can be confusing, and you may need some breastfeeding support to help you identify it. Resolving fussing due to slow flow can be as simple as swapping sides more frequently, increasing milk production or swapping the bottle teat to a faster flow.

Fast flow

Just as milk that is flowing too slowly can cause crying, so can milk which is flowing too fast. If milk is entering a baby's mouth too quickly, the baby may be unable to maintain a regular suck, swallow, breathe pattern. With fast flow we often see baby drinking and then suddenly start to choke, gasp, or cry. This is sometimes labelled as reflux since it happens so suddenly. Some babies will latch, suck and swallow several times and then unlatch to catch up on some breathing before repeating this pattern. Some babies might show more subtle signs of stress like furrowing their brow or splaying their fingers. Some babies might choke, unlatch and then seem to shut down and sleep for a short time before wanting to feed again. At the breast babies may seem happy before and between milk ejections, but you may see choking or crying during a milk ejection, or perhaps during the first milk ejection of each feed. The lack of a coordinated suck, swallow, breathe rhythm can lead to babies aspirating milk (milk going down the wrong way), or to swallowing air.

If breastfeeding, the resolution might be adjusting the positioning and attachment to help baby to manage the flow better, or adjusting milk supply to meet baby's needs better. If a baby is gaining weight very rapidly (approx 1lb or 450g a week in the first three months) there may be an oversupply of milk. This increased milk in the breast increases the pressure in the breast and so increases the rate of milk flow from the breast to baby's mouth when the baby sucks. If a breastfed baby is struggling with fast flow in combination with excessive weight gain, then adjusting the feeding pattern (by perhaps swapping sides less frequently than before) can reduce the volume of milk to match your baby's needs better and reduce the flow. This should be done cautiously and only if weight gain suggests that volume is an issue. I would suggest contacting an IBCLC or breastfeeding counsellor to talk this through.

If bottle-feeding, resolution might involve a slower flow teat, and/or carefully pacing bottle feeds.

If breastfeeding support or the changes to bottle-feeding don't help, an evaluation of swallowing from a speech and language therapist may be needed.

Tongue-tie

Tongue-tie is a condition which affects perhaps around 5% of babies.[4] In the womb the baby's developing tongue starts off fully fused to the floor of the mouth and as they grow and develop a process takes place which removes tissue and causes the tongue to become free from the floor of the mouth. This leaves a small membrane (frenulum) under the tongue which attaches the underside of the tongue to the floor of the mouth. In some babies this process doesn't seem to complete correctly and the frenulum attaches in a way that restricts movement of the tongue, or 'ties' the tongue.

This can affect reflux or cause what we commonly consider to be reflux symptoms in several ways. Firstly, a baby who has a tongue-tie or any issues with coordinating their tongue movement may have difficulty managing even normal flow and may cry during feeds and display the same kind of behaviour as we've described above in relation to fast flow. They may be simply unable to move their tongue in the way required to easily manage the flow of milk from front to back of the mouth, manage the swallow and protect the airway.

Secondly, tongue-tie may lead to a suboptimal latch on breast or bottle as the baby may be unable to open their mouth wide and extend their tongue to contact and cup the breast or bottle teat, and then create a wave-like motion to suckle. This may lead to a shallow latch, chewing, leaking milk and a poor suck and swallow pattern, all of which may also lead to frustration, or choking and crying during feeds.

If bottle-feeding, the caregiver may be able to manage the feeds through careful pacing and positioning of the bottle, but in my experience most bottle-feeding parents are not supported to recognise what is normal feeding and when a baby is having problems with feeding. Certainly with the families I see, weight gain appears to be the primary concern of healthcare professionals. Whereas a baby may be able to chew or latch shallowly on a bottle without anyone noticing a problem (other than perhaps very slow feedings), a baby doing the same at the breast usually causes pain and trauma for the breastfeeding mother, and this may further reduce the amount of milk a baby gets.

All of these difficulties with tongue movement can lead to an altered feeding pattern. A tongue-tied baby who is breastfeeding may rely on a high milk supply to help them drink. This can lead to a baby wanting to swap sides very frequently, getting high volumes of milk in a short time, which can lead to more spit up due to the volume of milk. Other babies will spend long periods of time at the breast getting very little milk and having very poor weight gain, and this may lead to arching and crying due to hunger. This is often misinterpreted as wind or silent reflux.

On a bottle it may lead to very slow feeding times, bottle refusal and babies only taking small amounts and then giving up, leading to poor weight gain.

If tongue-tie is suspected, there needs to be a careful tongue assessment done by a trained healthcare professional or IBCLC and referral made to a tongue-tie practitioner to have the tie released. This involves a minor procedure to allow the tongue to move correctly.

Allergy and food hypersensitivity

Food hypersensitivity is quite commonly seen in babies suffering from GORD and may actually be responsible for the pain of reflux. In Chapter 2 we discussed how reflux does not cause pain to the healthy oesophagus, but where there is damage to the oesophagus already, reflux can enter the cells and trigger pain receptors. Potentially this can also happen when drinking milk and the milk is touching damaged tissue. Some babies certainly seem to be very uncomfortable when feeding, even when latched well and managing the flow. Some refuse milk. Some take very small amounts and their weight falters. If your baby is not gaining weight the first step is to see your doctor and an IBCLC if breastfeeding. If medical issues and latch and suck issues are ruled out and there are other signs of allergy present, your care provider may discuss the possibility of food hypersensitivity with you.

Other signs of allergy may include:

- Skin rashes
- Hives
- Eczema
- Swelling (particularly around the lips, face and eyes)
- Nausea
- Abdominal pain
- Constipation or diarrhoea
- Blood or mucous in stools
- Redness around the anus
- Fatigue

Food hypersensitivity is also more likely if there is a family history of allergy. If a baby is having feeding issues in conjunction with some of the signs above then food allergy should be investigated. The most common food allergy in babies is cow's milk, followed by eggs, but potentially we can be sensitised and become allergic to any food.

For a formula-feeding baby, allergy to dairy will involve being prescribed an amino acid formula, or moving to breastfeeding (through relactation or donor milk). For a breastfeeding baby, food allergy usually requires the breastfeeding mother to eliminate that food from their diet. Once the allergen is removed, and the body heals and inflammation reduces, any reflux should become normal, non-painful reflux.

Crying after feeding
The acid reflux theory of GORD assumes that TLOSRs which occur after a feed allow acid to contact the oesophagus and cause pain and crying. In my experience there can be many reasons for crying after feeds which aren't due to GORD.

Sometimes the reason can be as simple as too little or too much milk in that feed. If too much milk, a baby may feel relief from spitting up and then settle afterwards. Thickeners and alginates can prevent spitting up and can actually make a baby feel more uncomfortable. If this is happening, the solution would be to try smaller feeds more regularly and then reassess reflux symptoms.

If a baby is crying after a feed because they are still hungry they will likely settle when given more milk. When bottle-feeding it is easy to see how much milk a baby is drinking. Breastfeeding mothers, however, need to learn to identify when their baby is feeding well, perhaps watching for swallowing, learning to identify milk ejections and the change in sucking pattern or looking for the 'milk drunk' phase after a feed. If feeding is not going well, and a baby is not getting enough milk, they may unlatch and cry. Putting the baby back to the breast may not settle the baby if there is not enough milk in the breast, and this can lead to the mother feeling that the baby doesn't want more milk and is crying for some other reason – potentially due to silent reflux. If this is happening the clue will be in weight gain as your baby will likely have lower than average weight gain, and the steps to resolve would be to increase weight gain and then reassess the reflux symptoms.

Crying after feeding can also occur with food sensitivity, and in this situation a baby with normal reflux may have pain, whereas a baby with a healthy oesophagus could have the same reflux with no pain at all. Where allergy is an issue, other symptoms are usually present.

Babies may also cry after feeds if they are put down to sleep, simply because they are not being held, or because they still want to comfort suck.

Back arching during feeding

We've already discussed that a baby may back arch when the flow is too fast, or too slow, or they are having problems with attaching or maintaining a good latch on the breast or bottle. A newborn doesn't have a very large number of gross motor movements that they can do. The movements that they can make with their core muscles are essentially to arch back or to fold in (the two big movements of the core) and they may do these for a variety of reasons.

As well as arching in response to a problem with flow or wanting to swap sides at the breast, babies will also arch for other reasons. They may need to burp. They may even need to pee. In fact, families who use elimination communication with their baby (a method where rather than using nappies, the caregivers watch the baby for cues of needing to pee or poo and hold the baby over the toilet) often see arching or popping on and off the breast as a signal that the baby needs to use the toilet.

Arching during feeds in and of itself wouldn't be a diagnostic symptom of GORD as it can be a symptom of many other feeding issues.

When discussing arching it is also worthwhile discussing arching during sleep or when laid down. Some babies appear to arch when laid flat, and/or may hold their head to one side. Parents often worry about this being a symptom of Sandifer's syndrome. The theory is that the baby is extending their oesophagus as much as possible in order to prevent reflux reaching the mouth. In reality Sandifer's syndrome is rare. However, postural issues which need time and/or therapy to resolve are common in newborns. Babies can be very squashed in the pelvis in the last few weeks of pregnancy. Some babies may not be positioned perfectly. Some may even be in a breech or transverse position for a long time, for example. The uterus is a shaped container and a baby's body and skull are quite malleable during pregnancy and in early infancy. This is by design, to allow the baby to fit through the birth canal. This malleability means that the position that a baby is in for many weeks in the uterus can mould the baby, as can instruments such as forceps or vacuum used during birth. We will all have seen babies with very moulded heads after birth, or know of babies with moulded ankles and feet (positional talipes) or clicky hips which may need treatment. A study in 2008 found that over 10% of babies have some kind of moulding, including plagiocephaly (flattening of the head) or torticollis (head tilted to the side).[5]

Head and body moulding can feed into arching in a few ways. A baby with a moulded head or body may not be in an optimal position when feeding, or may have some asymmetry around their mouth leading to a poor latch at either breast or bottle, and potentially poor tongue movement. Any thorough feeding assessment should look at any postural asymmetries.

Comfort feeding or frequent feeding

Babies who feed frequently or feed for long periods of time are sometimes assumed to be comfort feeding in order to reduce the pain of reflux. For a Western society which may have a skewed idea of what is normal feeding (3–4-hourly feeds), a baby who is actually feeding in a normal pattern may be incorrectly labelled as comfort feeding, so it's important to assess feeding against biological norms. It's also important to assess the feeding time in context of the overall picture. A baby who is feeding for an hour at a time, with a very short gap before starting again, and who has low weight gain is not comfort feeding, but is clearly having difficulty feeding. A baby who is feeding in this pattern and is gaining within the normal range also needs feeding carefully assessed. This pattern is usually not due to GORD, but to some feeding difficulty around getting enough milk in a normal timeframe. This might be due to flow rate, volume or difficulty in managing the suck, swallow, breathe rhythm.

It's also important to consider the physiological need to suckle. Very young babies need to suckle, and time spent suckling isn't always about milk. It can also be about body regulation.

Babies do often want to comfort feed after spitting up, but that doesn't necessarily mean they have GORD. It might be more about the taste of the milk, or refilling the tummy or relaxing the nervous system.

Poor weight gain

When silent reflux is queried one of the first questions I always ask is about weight gain. Babies who are not getting enough milk will be hungry and unsettled. Hungry babies will cry, not sleep well, not want to be put down, and exhibit colicky behaviour. With a bottle it is easy to see if a baby has drunk the expected amount of milk and is still hungry, but it is less easy when breastfeeding. A breastfed baby may arch at the breast, be unsettled and have low weight gain if the baby isn't getting enough milk. These symptoms taken together, without a good feeding assessment, may lead to a diagnosis of silent reflux.

If a baby has low weight gain the first step is to increase calorie intake. In almost all babies this will resolve the weight gain.

My baby spent the entire time between feeds wincing and crying. He was bringing something up between feeds, then squealing and crying... After feeding on both sides

– a real noticeable difference. Feeding is going so much better. Annemarie

If a baby is not gaining well despite adequate calorie intake the baby should be investigated for any medical issues causing an issue with weight intake. If there are allergy symptoms alongside the low weight gain, allergy should be investigated.

High weight gain

High weight gain alongside unsettled behaviour can also sometimes be attributed to reflux. The theory is that the baby is feeding so frequently to soothe the reflux that the excessive intake causes the high weight gain. In my experience the relationship is more commonly the other way around. It's not that reflux causes the high weight gain, but rather that very high weight gain can cause reflux symptoms. Average weight gain for a baby in the first three months is around 8oz a week. A baby who is gaining closer to 1lb each week may have excessive spit up from the volume of milk, may arch during feeds due to the volume of milk and may have colicky crying and gas due to the volume of lactose (milk sugar) in the gut. If reflux is suspected in a baby who has very high weight gain (approximately double the average) it may be worthwhile reducing intake slightly and then reassessing symptoms. Any reduction in intake should be discussed with your lactation consultant or the baby's care provider.

Unsettled behaviours

Excessive crying

Excessive crying is often listed as a diagnostic indicator of GORD – again the theory is that acid reflux causes pain and thus crying. In this section I want to look more closely at the definition of *excessive* crying. How do we know if a baby is crying excessively?

How much crying is normal? Here, I'm going to draw from research on colic, as colic is often defined as excessive crying in a baby who is otherwise healthy and thriving. A commonly used measure in colic is Wessel's criteria or the 'rule of 3s', which is crying for at least three hours a day, for at least three days a week for at least three weeks in a row. This is a useful measure as it describes a pattern of sustained, ongoing crying over a period of time, whereas a baby who is unwell due to a bug or is unsettled during a growth spurt is unlikely to meet the three weeks criteria.

Research suggests that around 5% of babies meet the rule of 3s definition of excessive crying.[6] If your baby does fall into this category you should certainly discuss the excessive crying with your GP and have a feeding assessment from someone qualified in assessing feeding to rule out any of the feeding issues already discussed as well as potential underlying medical conditions. Parenting a baby with colic, where there is sustained crying over weeks and months, is extremely difficult and requires a lot of support. We don't know what causes true colic. Some theories suggest there may be gut distress which may cause headaches, but a very interesting theory suggests that it is a temporary glitch in the development of 'speech breathing' and not related to pain at all. There is more on this in Chapter 8.

Many of the babies who are diagnosed with GORD do not meet the rule of 3s and are often described as 'colicky' rather than being diagnosed as having colic. Often these babies are either crying around feeding, or having a fussy crying period in the evenings. Any baby who is crying during or after feeding is potentially having a feeding issue and should have feeding assessed to see if this is a cause of crying. As before, too fast flow, too slow flow, poor latch, poor suck, swallow, breathe sequence and so on can all cause crying during feeds and are not indicative of reflux but of a feeding issue. Fussy periods in the evening also need to be assessed in the context of the larger picture. If a baby is content during the morning and early afternoon, and happy sleeping in your arms during dark hours, but unhappy in the evening or unhappy sleeping alone, is this really indicating reflux? Why would reflux be causing pain only in the evening or at times the baby is alone, but not during the day? If a baby lies on their back in your arms contentedly, but not on their back in a cot, is this really a sign of GORD, or of a baby who is asking to be held? And if a baby is unsettled for a period each night, is this reflux, or is it the well-known fussy evenings or 'witching hours' that babies commonly have? Or could it be evening intestinal gas, which isn't a symptom of GORD?

'She woke up crying every time I set her down and I assumed it was reflux. As I held my baby more and kept her close for sleep, she became more settled.' Melanie

Some level of crying is unfortunately quite normal in the first three months of life. Even when babies are held or carried virtually all the time, and are responded to promptly, they still cry sometimes, because this is the only way they can verbally get our attention. Babies are communicating with us right from the beginning, but if we are unable to distinguish their non-verbal cues (and it takes us a few weeks to learn them), then they need to communicate their needs to us by crying. We'll look at infant communication in more detail in Chapter 8.

Waking often at night

Just like excessive crying, whether frequent waking is a cause for concern can only be assessed by looking at it in the context of normal waking, and what our expectations of night sleep and night waking are for a baby. In WEIRD societies (Western, Educated, Industrialised, Rich, Democratic) there is often quite a skewed idea of what normal infant sleep is. We tend to have an idea of normal sleep for an adult to be eight hours of uninterrupted sleep and we expect babies to move towards this pattern as soon as possible, and often to more like 10–12 hours of uninterrupted sleep. Varying too much from this expectation is often categorised as 'bad' sleep. It doesn't help that new parents often get a stream of questions from friends, relatives and complete strangers about whether their baby is a 'good sleeper'. Setting aside the fact that eight uninterrupted hours may not even be a normal biological pattern for an adult, babies have different sleep needs and different sleep patterns from an adult, which can take significant time to mature.

When we sleep we sleep in cycles. These cycles include falling asleep, dream sleep, light sleep and deep sleep, and then back up through these stages of deep sleep, light sleep, dream sleep and then a brief awakening before moving into the next cycle and repeating the stages. We do this each night. Adults' sleep cycles are approximately 90 minutes long and all of us, adults and children, briefly wake after each cycle. We may turn over, adjust the pillow or sheets, or just go straight back to sleep, usually not remembering anything about it in the morning.

Babies have much shorter sleep cycles, and young babies aren't able to turn over or adjust their sleeping environment. They often need a little help to get into the next sleep cycle. A newborn has a sleep cycle of around 45 minutes, and an eight-month-old about 50 minutes, so it doesn't suddenly change at three or six months when some books suggest that babies should be sleeping long stretches.[7] No babies sleep for hours without waking. They will all have brief awakenings between sleep cycles. Some babies are able to move into a new sleep cycle more easily than others and this may be personality based as much as anything. Some of us are more relaxed than others, while some of us are more anxious. Some of us fall asleep easily and sleep all night, and some of us toss and turn. Some of us can fall asleep in cars, on planes and in new situations, and some of us don't fall asleep easily unless we are in our own beds at home. Even when relaxed on holiday some of us don't sleep well in the first couple of days simply because it is a new environment in which our body doesn't feel totally safe. In adults none of this is related to GORD, and the same is true for babies. It's often about our feelings of stress or safety.

Frequent waking is in fact protective for small babies. Newborns have a very immature nervous system and that includes their respiration system, which is why young babies are vulnerable to SIDS. Frequent waking is part of the protection against SIDS, and this frequent waking is actually the solution to the dangers of deep continual sleep for a baby. Thinking of it this way can help us approach night wake-ups differently.

It is normal for newborns to wake every 2–3 hours during the night for feeds. Many may take a longer stretch between feeds, but equally many do not. Research suggests that at three months 58% of babies are sleeping a five-hour stretch from 12–5am.[8] At four months 58% are sleeping an eight-hour stretch. At five months 53% are sleeping for eight hours. All of these figures are pretty close to 50:50, meaning it is normal if your baby is not sleeping these long stretches – after all, half the baby population isn't! The other thing that is clear from these figures is that sleep development is not linear. Stretches of sleep do not automatically get longer and longer as a baby gets older. The research I've quoted here shows us that fewer babies are sleeping for eight hours at five months than at three or four months. Sleep development is not a straight line. Awakenings increase and decrease at different times over the first year.

So babies are meant to wake frequently and it is protective. They need to feed frequently and they need to have a lot of nervous system regulation from a mature adult nervous system (i.e. be held, rocked and soothed). The problem is that we as adults have created a society in which we are unable to sleep frequently during the day (as babies do). Even in societies where a siesta is common, such as Spain, the afternoon nap is becoming less common than it used to be. We have created a situation in which we need to get almost all our sleep requirements in one night-time burst. We complicate this further by drinking caffeine during the day and evening and by using phones and devices which shine light into our eyes at all hours of the day and night, even sometimes during night feeds. We know that this behaviour affects sleep. In fact, ingesting caffeine in the six hours before we sleep reduces our overall night-time sleep hours, and the light from devices disrupts our light/dark cycle and reduces our sleep.[9] This means that for most of us it is the parents who have the sleep problem. We need to find ways to get more sleep in each 24-hour period, rather than expecting our babies to sleep more like adults. Sleep deprivation can be brutal for our mental health, and affect our ability to function well or to enjoy our babies, so it is totally understandable that we search for fixes. The first year of parenting is very difficult sleep-wise even if a baby is entirely well, healthy and free of GORD.

A baby with GORD is generally unsettled for much of the

day and night. The disturbance is rarely just at night. If you are worried about GORD, think about your sleep environment and when your baby is unsettled. Is your baby just as unsettled in someone's arms? Are they just as unsettled if they are on their tummy against someone's chest or shoulder? Would they sleep better there? If so, does that fit with GORD, or does it fit with a baby who is communicating a need to be held? Could it be that their need to be held is something you hadn't anticipated but is normal? Could the waking be normal frequent waking? Could your baby be going through a growth spurt (which often leads to much more frequent waking)?

Colicky or windy

A baby is often described as 'colicky' if they are very unsettled but don't meet the Wessel criteria for colic. Colicky crying in a young baby is often attributed to wind. Wind is a catch-all term, interchangeably used to describe air in the stomach causing a need to burp, and also for digestive gas in the gastrointestinal tract and the need to pass that gas.

Digestive gas

Let's start with the gastrointestinal (GI) tract and digestive gas. Gas in the GI tract is primarily caused by digestion of foods by bacteria in the bowel. When babies are born they have very few bacteria in the GI tract. Adults, in contrast, are estimated to have as many bacterial cells in their body as human cells, and the vast majority of these bacteria are in and around the gut.[10] These colonies of bacteria in the gut are known as the gut microbiota, and our microbiota is very important for healthy digestion and even healthy immune function. A baby needs to set up these bacterial colonies and a lot of this colonisation takes place in the weeks after birth. This takes place from the environment (e.g. from contact with other people, animals, things they touch or put in their mouths) and from what a baby eats and drinks.

During the early weeks the gut is becoming colonised and those colonising bacteria are digesting food, creating gas as part of their digestion, multiplying in numbers, digesting more food, creating more gas and multiplying in numbers. When you consider this ongoing, increasing process it makes sense that babies are windy. It's estimated that adults create 0.6–1.8 litres of gas a day, and release that gas 12–25 times a day.[11] Part of what helps us to release that gas is movement. Movement helps with gut motility, but small babies often move very little. They are often in cots, chairs, prams and strollers for a lot of the day.

Many people find that when their baby is on their tummy, either in tummy time on the floor, or on a caregiver's shoulder or breast, they pass gas more easily. Many people find that when breastfeeding their baby burps more easily too. It may be that the baby has pressure on their tummy that they can move against (like a self-massage), or it may be that they are more relaxed in that tummy position because they feel more stable, and because they are more relaxed all functions of digestion work better.

I suspect every adult has had painful gas at some stage and knows how uncomfortable it is. For a small baby who is struggling to pass gas, infant massage can be extremely helpful to encourage gut motility. There is no doubt that gas can be painful, but it isn't a diagnostic indicator of GORD.

Babies who are drinking very large volumes of milk (much larger than average) can experience excess gas due to the levels of sugar in the milk. The main sugar in milk is lactose. This sugar is broken down by an enzyme in the intestine called lactase. If a baby gets too much milk overall, or takes a very large feed (so has too much milk at one time) the intestine receives a huge dose of lactose, and is just not able to produce enough lactase to digest it all. This produces symptoms very similar to lactose intolerance, but it is actually a case of lactose overwhelm. In this situation, not all of the lactose can be broken down and some makes it to the colon undigested. The colon is the area of the GI tract which is teeming with the bacteria mentioned above, and now we have provided them with lots of sugar to digest. That digestion leads to a lot of gas in the colon, and may lead to pain/discomfort from that gas. If this is the case, then normalising milk intake resolves the excess gas and the discomfort.

'I've been block feeding to reduce his milk and many of the reflux symptoms have cleared up.' Tamsin

Swallowed air when feeding

Gas also comes from being swallowed. If air is swallowed and isn't released back out through the mouth or nose in a burp it can be passed from the stomach through to the intestine. This means that a baby who is swallowing a lot of air while feeding can have excessive gas. However, a baby who is feeding well, coordinating the flow of milk well and drinking an appropriate amount at each feed should not be taking in much air. I have searched for research on swallowing air while feeding from bottles, and although society worries a lot about this problem, I found little research to support the idea that it is an issue. We do have some ultrasound research looking at babies feeding from the breast, and from this we find no evidence of large amounts of air being swallowed when a baby is feeding well.[12] Certainly, for decades there has been a belief that bottles cause air to be swallowed, which is why we have a myriad of bottles with different air valve solutions. It's only in recent years, however, that we've had a better understanding of the need to carefully pace bottle-feeds. Traditionally there has been a societal view that babies should drink large volumes of milk at each feed and that they should drink that milk through a fast-flow teat and therefore quickly. Parents are rarely taught how to identify the signs of a baby being stressed by the speed of the milk flow. In fact I have seen parents misidentify stress signs (finger splaying) as a sign that their baby was loving the fast flow. Babies who are not managing the flow of milk well and are stressed by it may have a mismanaged suck, swallow, breathe process, which may lead to more air being swallowed. So a baby who is suspected of swallowing air while feeding should have their feeding carefully assessed. If large amounts of air are being swallowed while feeding, there is a feeding issue.

Abdominal pressure when crying

One study, looking at the effects of crying in babies, describes it as follows: *'A cry is a series of four movements that basically resembles a Valsalva maneuver.'* [13]

If you aren't familiar with a Valsalva manoeuvre, it is the move we sometimes do to help our ears to pop when we are in an aeroplane, where we close our mouth, hold our nose closed and breathe out hard, increasing the pressure in our chest and head. It increases blood pressure, decreases oxygen, increases heart rate and also increases abdominal pressure. If you try a Valsalva manoeuvre you will notice that you tense your abdominal muscles. You may have noticed a tense, tight tummy on your baby when they cry. During research reflux has been found to be more likely to occur during crying due to the increased pressure. [14] It may be that a crying baby is suspected to be crying due to painful reflux, when in fact the reflux may be due to crying. Reducing our baby's crying by more responsive care and body contact for much of the day may reduce reflux.

Abdominal pressure from constipation

Crying isn't the only thing to increase abdominal pressure. Straining to pass a bowel motion also causes increased abdominal pressure, and straining will be increased by constipation. Even without straining, constipation makes reflux more likely. A full rectum causes the stomach to empty more slowly through a mechanism called the cologastric brake.[15]

Vomiting, nausea, bloating and stomach pain are commonly seen in people with constipation, and relieving the constipation can be the factor that resolves the vomiting/nausea and other stomach symptoms. A 2004 study looking at children with nausea and reflux found that their reflux resolved entirely when the constipation was treated.[16]

A baby under six weeks old should move their bowels daily at least once (but likely several times every day). A baby under six weeks old may even have a dirty nappy for every feed. Any baby under six weeks old who is not moving their bowels daily should have their feeding evaluated as the most common reason is not drinking enough milk (which will likely also cause crying).

After six weeks the majority of babies do have fewer dirty nappies. Some babies may only have a day or two between movements, while some might go as long as 10–15 days. The weekly or 10-day pattern may be described to you as normal, and may be considered statistically normal, but it may not necessarily be physiologically normal. Parents of breastfed babies are often told that breastmilk leaves no waste and therefore it is fine for their baby to poo infrequently, but this isn't backed up by what we know about breastmilk. The third most abundant component in breastmilk is special milk sugars called human milk oligosaccharides (HMOs). HMOs cannot be digested by babies and appear to be in milk solely in order to facilitate bacteria in the gut.[17] These sugars are not all used up by the baby. Poo contains old cells which slough off from the intestinal lining, bile, old blood cells and so on. None of these things are 'used up'. In fact, babies who are pooing infrequently tend to have a massive movement every few days. This suggests that the poo was actually sitting in the bowel for several days and simply wasn't moving out.

Although some breastfed babies have days between stooling, most are still having daily dirty nappies. If breastmilk is all used up, then how could this be the case? How could some babies drinking breastmilk be creating waste and others not? In the book *Baby Poop: What Your Paediatrician May Not Tell You* (p182), Linda Palmer writes:

> 'Some exclusively breastfed babies will go 7 to 10 days, and dare I say even 17 days between poops, without having hard or painful stools. This is common enough that most doctors call it normal. In my experience, any such baby I've worked with has had some other issues going on and has benefitted from working through these issues. You may like to think of it like constipation, in terms of searching for causes, especially when it regularly goes beyond three days'.[18]

PART II

Resolving Reflux

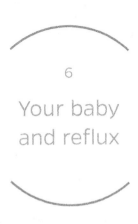

6

Your baby
and reflux

Part II of this book is designed to help you work through your baby's reflux symptoms systematically to help determine whether your baby may have normal infant reflux, which management techniques may be helpful, and whether your baby may have GORD. The steps here are intended to help guide you through working out what might be normal baby behaviour or abnormal behaviour, and is informed by evidence-based research, but it cannot be taken as a diagnosis. Any diagnosis of GORD can only come from your baby's doctor.

Step 1: Your baby's symptoms
Start by making a list of your baby's symptoms. Write down everything that makes you worry about reflux.

Step 2: Check your baby's weight gain
Make a note of your baby's weight gain over the last few

weeks. If your baby is being weighed infrequently, average the weight over the last few weeks. For example, if your baby is four weeks old and the last weight check was two weeks ago, divide the weight gain by two to get the average weekly gain.

Weight check

Average weight gain for a baby under 12 weeks is around 7-8oz/200–220g a week

- Less than 5oz/140g a week is low weight gain
- Over 12oz/340g a week is high weight gain
- Between 5oz/140g and 12oz/340g a week is normal weight gain

Average weight gain for a baby over 12 weeks is around 4-5oz/120–150g

- Less than 3oz/90g a week is low weight gain
- Over 8oz/230g a week is high weight gain
- Between 3oz/90g and 8oz/230g is normal weight gain

The most common reason for either low or high weight gain is the amount of milk calories a baby is getting. This means that the most likely reason for low weight gain is that your baby is not drinking enough milk each day. The most likely reason for high weight gain is that your baby is drinking a high volume of milk each day.

Milk intake increases rapidly over the first few weeks of life. In the first 2–3 days a baby is designed to drink small amounts of colostrum, but the volumes increase quite rapidly after the first couple of days. Average intake for a breastfed baby in the first few days is as follows:

Day 1	7ml per feed
Day 2	14ml per feed
Day 3	30–50ml per feed
Day 4	50–70ml per feed

By day 7 a breastfed baby is drinking around 600ml (21oz) a day on average.[1,2]

A formula feeding baby will get larger volumes right from day 1, and will likely be taking 30–50ml immediately.

By 2–3 weeks we expect a baby to be drinking 60–90ml (2–3oz) in each feed. By 3–4 weeks we expect that volume to be around 90–120ml (3–4oz) per feed. Babies should feed at least eight times a day, so at 3–4 weeks the overall volume might be around 750–800ml (25–28oz) per day. By 5–6 weeks a baby may be taking anything between 750–1,000ml (25–35oz) a day with an average of 800ml (28oz).

If your baby has low weight gain – read Box A
If your baby has high weight gain – read Box B
If your baby has normal weight gain – Go to Step 3

BOX A: My baby has low weight gain

Work on normalising weight gain, as low weight gain can cause unsettledness, crying and difficult feeding behaviours such as back arching or fussiness while feeding.

If you are breastfeeding

Seek support around increasing milk intake/increasing milk supply. This may involve improving positioning and attachment, switching sides more frequently and feeding more frequently. It may also involve expressing and supplementing for a period of time. Consider the statements below to help you assess your feeding:

- My baby rouses easily for feeds and feeds actively.
- I can tell the difference between sucking and swallowing.
- I can tell when I have a milk ejection/letdown.
- My baby is getting 2–4 milk ejections at each feed.

If you have answered no to any of the above questions, ask your breastfeeding supporter to help you identify swallowing and milk ejections so that you can use this to assess feeds going forward. An IBCLC, breastfeeding counsellor or appropriately trained healthcare professional can help with this.

If you are bottle-feeding
Seek support about the volumes of milk your baby needs in each bottle and how frequently your baby should be feeding at this stage. As a general guideline a baby needs around 150ml for every kg of body weight over a 24-hour period. This means that a 4kg baby needs 600ml (150 x 4) every 24 hours. This should be over at least eight feeds, but may be more than eight.

No matter how you feed
General guidelines to help increase intake are:

1. Feed more frequently. Rather than feeding every three hours, try offering a feed every two hours. This may suit your baby better and will fit in 1–2 extra feeds over the course of the day. Many babies prefer to drink smaller amounts more frequently,

and this may reduce levels of vomit.

2. Feed responsively. If your baby cues for a feed or seems unsettled before the 2–3 hour mark, offer a feed.

3. If your baby is very sleepy, ensure that you wake your baby so that there are at least eight feeds a day.

4. When working out how often your baby is feeding, count the time from the start of a feed to the start of the next feed. Sometimes it can be hard to count the number of feeds, particularly if a baby is cluster feeding, and babies who aren't getting enough milk often have very sleepy, frequent feeds. If your baby feeds, falls asleep and then goes back to the breast within 20 minutes, count it as the same feed. If there is at least a 20-minute break, count it as a new feed.

5. Reduce the use of dummies/pacifiers. Sucking on a dummy raises levels of a hormone called CCK which makes a baby feel full and can then reduce the amount of milk they drink.[3] Rather than offering a dummy, try offering another feed.

If you have put the above steps in place, are certain that your baby is getting enough milk for their weight/age and they are still not gaining within normal range, see your doctor to assess your baby's wellbeing, as some medical conditions can cause a higher than normal calorie need.

Once weight gain has normalised, repeat Step 1 and reassess your baby's reflux symptoms to see if they have changed.

BOX B: My baby has high weight gain

Work on normalising weight gain by normalising milk intake volume. High milk intake can cause excessive gas, crying and fussy feeding.

If you are breastfeeding
Seek support around reducing milk intake at the breast in a managed way that still allows your baby to comfort suck when they need. This might involve using cold compresses on your breasts after a feed to slow milk production, swapping sides less frequently, or even using a dummy at times.

If you are bottle-feeding
Seek support around the volume needed for your baby in each bottle. Slow the flow of milk from the bottle so that your baby does not overfeed. Use paced feeding techniques, watching carefully for signs of stress (see Chapter 7). Try covering the bottle when you are feeding so that you don't notice whether there is milk left in the bottle. This reduces the temptation to encourage your baby to finish the bottle.

Once weight gain has normalised, repeat Step 1 and reassess your baby's reflux symptoms to see if they have changed.

Step 3: My baby's feeding behaviours
When assessing this stage you will have already worked through the weight gain stage and know that your baby's weight gain is in normal range. Now look at the symptoms

you listed in Step 1 and work through the relevant boxes below.

My baby is spitting up a lot

Check how frequently your baby is feeding. Count this from start of a feed until the start of the next feed.

My baby feeds:
- Less than two-hourly on average
- 2–3 hourly on average
- 3–4 hourly on average
- More than four-hourly on average

If your baby is feeding 3–4 hourly or more, try offering smaller feeds more frequently.

If bottle-feeding

Rather than six feeds of 5–6 oz/150–180ml, try 8–10 feeds of 3–4oz/(90–120ml. Use paced feeding techniques to help your baby take the feed more slowly and become more satisfied with smaller volumes.

No matter how you feed

1. If your baby is not distressed by the vomit, or initially becomes upset but settles easily after spitting up, reassess the behaviour against the information in this book to work out whether it could just be a laundry problem rather than GORD.

2. Use upright positions after feeds and create optimal digestion by increasing body contact and keeping your baby against you. Consider using slings between feeds and for some daytime sleeps so that

your baby has body contact for most of the day.

3. If your baby has persistent projectile vomiting (the vomit lands several feet away) see your doctor to check for any medical conditions.

4. If your baby is constipated (regularly not stooling on a daily basis) work on helping your baby become more regular at stooling. Straining due to constipation increases abdominal pressure and this can lead to more vomiting. Regular tummy time, tummy massage and body contact can help. If this is not enough, talk to your doctor about a gentle laxative.

5. If vomiting is constant (small possets every few minutes all day long) and you are breastfeeding, think about whether there are any LOS looseners in your diet (see Chapter 4, pp. 64-5), and whether reducing these could help.

My baby cries or back arches during a feed

Back arching can have multiple causes. Pick the scenarios which fit for your baby:

1. *My breastfed baby wants to feed but then cries/fusses within a few seconds of starting a feed.*
   Observe the next few feeds to see if there is a pattern. Does your baby pop off and on the breast crying for a couple of minutes but then settle and feed well (during the letdown/milk ejection)? Is the fussing less of an issue in the morning when your breasts are fuller? Is it more of an issue in the

evenings when your breasts are emptier? Does your baby pull or tug on your nipple? If so, your baby may be frustrated by slow flow at the start of the feed. Breast compressions may help. Seek support around whether increasing your milk supply may also help as fuller breasts have faster milk flow.

2. *My breastfed baby is content at the start of a feed but then becomes upset during my letdown/milk ejection.*

   Seek breastfeeding support around helping your baby to manage your letdown. Changing your position to use more laid-back or side-lying positions may help your baby to cope better as they will be more stable and have better tongue movement. Getting a deeper attachment may also help your baby to manage the flow better. If your baby comes off the breast and you notice your milk spraying, let it spray into a muslin cloth or small container and then relatch your baby when the flow slows. Check if you are feeling stressed, and if so, try some relaxation techniques. Relaxing your body will help your baby relax and that will help with sucking coordination.

3. *My breastfed baby is content for the first five minutes of a feed and then starts to fuss and cry.*

   Research tells us that a breast can be 50% emptied after just five minutes, and once the breast starts to empty milk flow slows down. Babies can be fussy when the flow slows as it is harder to get the milk. This is frustrating for a hungry baby. Breast compressions may help your baby get some faster flow, but if your baby still seems fussy then they may be asking to switch sides. Try switching to see if your baby settles with the faster milk flow on the other side. It is ok to switch back and forth, and many people do this in the evenings when babies are fussier.

4. *My bottle-fed baby is happy for the first half of the feed and then becomes very upset and doesn't want the rest of the bottle.*

    Reassess the frequency of feeds and the volume in each feed. Could your baby be asking for smaller volumes more frequently? Could you have missed some early stress cues, or cues that your baby wanted a break or had had enough milk for now? Use more frequent paced feeding.

5. *My baby seems to be struggling when feeding. Milk leaks from the sides of their mouth or they seem to chew or clamp down on the bottle teat or on the breast.*

    Check how your baby is latched to the bottle or breast.

    If breastfeeding
    Seek support around positioning and attachment. Breast shaping may help your baby to latch on more deeply and to stay attached. If the flow of milk seems too fast for your baby then using laid-back positions may help.

    If bottle-feeding
    Check the shape of your baby's teat and whether your baby's lips are well down the neck of the teat. If you find your baby's lips are close to the nipple of the teat, you may find that a narrower teat suits your baby better. Try paced bottle-feeding techniques to help your baby to control the flow of

milk. If your baby continues to struggle regardless of these changes, you may want to have your baby evaluated for tongue-tie.

6. *My baby seems to be in pain when feeding. I can hear gas in my baby's tummy, and their tummy is hard.*
   Review whether your baby may have gas due to high milk intake, or whether your baby may be constipated. If neither of these are the case, see Step 4 on unsettled behaviour.

7. *My baby seems to be in pain when milk touches their throat, and is refusing feeds much of the time.*
   Read through the sections in the book about fast flow to assess whether your baby may be struggling with managing the flow. Seek support from an IBCLC or other infant feeding specialist to assess the feed. Complete Step 3 looking at allergy.

8. *I feel anxious during feeds because I am worried about my baby's feeding and about reflux.*
   Your baby may be picking up on your anxiety and this will make your baby more anxious too. A baby who feels stressed and anxious does not feed as well and this may be leading to a vicious cycle around feeding. Try conscious relaxation techniques before and during feeds.

My baby cries after a feed

1. *My baby cries immediately after a feed.*
   Assess how well your baby is managing the flow of the feed. Is your baby's body relaxed during a feed, and does your baby stop the feed themselves? If your baby is not relaxed and calm during the feed,

consider the flow of the milk. Observe a few feeds and look at your baby's swallowing pattern. If your baby is fussy during the feed and not swallowing much and cries immediately after the feed, your baby may be asking for more milk and the feed may not be finished.

If breastfeeding
Consider whether swapping sides more frequently and breast compressions may help.

No matter how you feed
If your baby has been swallowing well during the feed, consider whether they may be overfull and feeling uncomfortable. Reassess feeding frequency and volume.

2. *My baby cries 1–2 hours after each feed, but isn't due another feed.*
   Consider whether your baby's natural feeding rhythm might be smaller, more frequent feeds. Does your baby settle with more milk at this time? Could it be that your baby is clustering some feeds closer together so that they can sleep a longer stretch later?

My baby is feeding constantly day and night

1. *My baby is feeding really frequently all day long – often hourly – but is sleepy when feeding and never seems satisfied after a feed. I'm worried about silent*

reflux and that baby needs to feed to soothe reflux pain.

This is more likely to be a breastfed baby – as you can see how much milk a bottle-fed baby is getting, but it is possible for some breastfed babies to get into a pattern of frequent feeding but not drinking much milk each time. When this happens a vicious cycle ensues.

2. *Baby doesn't drink much and falls asleep – baby wakes 20–30 minutes later and realises they are still hungry – the breast is still quite empty from the feed a short time ago.*

   This means that the milk flow is slower and milk is harder to remove – baby goes to the breast, but only drinks a small amount due to the breast being empty and falls asleep while sucking. Baby wakes 20–30 minutes later and realises they are still hungry... and so on.

   If this is happening, seek some breastfeeding support to increase milk flow and milk transfer at the breast so that your baby is taking larger amounts at the breast and becoming full after a feed. Then reassess reflux symptoms in Step 1.

Step 4: My baby is generally unsettled

This step is focused on unsettled behaviour outside of feeds. Having worked through steps 1 and 2, we know your baby is having a normal volume and frequency of feeds, and has normal weight gain, and in Step 3 we looked at how adjustments to feeding behaviour may help.

My baby is generally content in the day, but will not settle at night

1. *My baby will not sleep on their back.*
   Consider your baby's sleep arrangement. Could it be that your baby is wanting to be closer to you, and is not settling because they are not in your arms? If your baby was able to sleep in your arms all night, even if lying horizontally, would your baby sleep contentedly, only waking to feed at normal feeding intervals? If so, then the issue is more likely that your baby wants to be with you, and less likely to be GORD.

   If you are breastfeeding
   Read about safe co-sleeping/breastsleeping as this may help you both to get more rest and your baby may sleep contentedly beside you.

   No matter how you are feeding
   Holding your baby for longer before you put them down to sleep may help. Wait until your baby is in a very deep sleep, with limp limbs, before gently laying them down to sleep. Co-sleeper cots/cribs which attach to your bed can be helpful in minimising separation and helping your baby to stay asleep. It is okay to rock, sway and feed your baby to sleep. Your baby does not have to be laid down 'sleepy but awake'. Babies often need help to fall asleep.

2. *My baby wakes every time I put them in the cot/ crib and wants to feed again, and then vomits frequently.*

   If your baby feeds well, seems satisfied and falls asleep in your arms, but then wakes very shortly after being put down but settles easily in your arms or at the breast, the likelihood is that your baby does not actually need more milk, but is looking for you and your body. Babies expect to be close to their caregiver at night, and become stressed when placed away from them (even when asleep). If your baby feeds each time this happens they may become overfull and then vomit. This vomiting, in turn, may lead to them wanting to feed again and a vicious cycle can ensue. Sleeping close to your baby using a co-sleeper cot or bed-sharing (if you can do so safely) may help your baby to settle more easily. Keeping your baby in your arms after a feed until they are in a deep sleep (limp limbs) may help you to transfer them to a separate sleep space with a longer time before waking again.

3. *My baby cries when I burp them at night and I'm worried that it is reflux pain and they need to feed again to soothe the pain.*

   If your baby feeds well, settles, goes to sleep in your arms and only becomes unsettled when you burp them, it may be the action of burping which is unsettling them. Burping often wakes babies and it may be that your baby is wanting to drift off into a nice deep night-time sleep and the burping is preventing this, leading to your baby becoming frustrated and upset. Consider whether your baby really needs to be burped each time, or whether you can do it in a more gentle way. After a feed holding a baby upright against your body (over your shoulder) for a few minutes can help gently bring up any wind.

If bottle-feeding
Slowing the pace of the feed may help reduce the burping needed.

4. *How can I get any sleep? I'm exhausted and stressed.*
Young babies cause a lot of lost sleep for their caregivers. This is part of normal night-time parenting, but it can lead to exhaustion and anxiety about sleep. This is even more pronounced if your expectations of normal baby sleep differ dramatically from what your baby is doing. Read through Chapter 8, then reassess whether your baby is sleeping normally for a baby and whether your expectations were realistic. Adjusting expectations can reduce anxiety, even if it doesn't change the sleep. Creating a sleep environment where you are close to your baby may also help significantly. Working on relaxation techniques during the day may also help at night by reducing stress hormones overall and helping you to get to sleep more quickly at night between feeds.

If your baby is content during the day it's unlikely that your baby is suffering from GORD – which affects babies both day and night.

My baby is unsettled in the day but feeds and sleeps well at night

1. If your baby sleeps well at night and you are following safe sleep guidelines and placing your baby on their back it is unlikely that your baby is suffering from GORD.

2. Consider whether there is something different about the way you are feeding your baby at night. If you are breastfeeding, are you using a different feeding position and could this make a difference? Could you try this position during the day? If bottle-feeding, is there anything different about frequency/volume of bottles or the way the bottle is offered?

3. Consider whether your environment during the day might be loud or over-stimulating or whether you might be feeling a little anxious, stressed or worried about your baby during the day. Sometimes the reason that babies settle more easily at night is because the caregiver's body is more relaxed for night-time feeds (they have just woken out of a sleep and are still relaxed and sleepy). Creating a more relaxing environment during the day for both of you may help, as may working on relaxing your own nervous system during the day. Relaxation techniques can help, as can mindfulness or meditation. Using a phone app to help you relax for a few minutes here and there during the day can make a big difference. Using slings during the day so that your baby gets lots of body contact can also help your baby to relax and feel safe and calm.

My baby is crying/unsettled/unhappy most of the time or has other digestive symptoms

A baby who is unhappy most of the day is very difficult for everyone in the family. In this situation it is important that you see a doctor to rule out any medical issues which are causing your baby distress. If you know that your baby is otherwise healthy, and you have also worked through the previous steps, you will already have resolved any feeding issues. You will also have looked at your baby's environment and will be holding your baby as much as possible. If, after all of this, your baby is still very unsettled in your arms, or seems to need constant movement/distraction to keep them settled, then there may be some other kind of digestive distress. The points below work through things you could consider.

1. *Are there other digestive symptoms?*
   Is your baby stooling daily, or does your baby regularly skip days between stooling? Does your baby seem to have to strain in order to pass a stool? Constipation is linked to vomiting, and resolving constipation can also reduce vomiting and discomfort to normal levels.[4] Regular tummy massage can often help a baby to pass gas and stools, as can tummy time. In some cases probiotics can also be of help. If there are many days between stools on a regular basis you may want to talk to your GP about a laxative on a temporary basis to help your baby shift to a more regular pattern.

2. *Are stools and gas foul smelling?*
   Breastmilk stools in particular should not have an offensive smell. If you notice a change in smell, or you find your baby's stools foul smelling, this may be due to the types of bacteria in your baby's gut. Some of the bacteria which produce foul-smelling gas also create pain in the gut from that gas. In those cases probiotics may also be worth considering. Discuss this with your care provider.

3. *Are your baby's stools mucousy?*
   Do you notice mucous strings or jelly-like globs in your baby's stools? Some mucous is normal in stools, but if there is so much that you regularly notice it, your baby's gut may be producing excess mucous. This may be a sign of some gut irritation. This could be due to teething (swallowing saliva), a cold (swallowing mucous) or a tummy bug, or antibiotics or reacting to something in the milk. In the case of a breastfeeding mum this might be something in her diet, or in a formula-fed baby it may be something in the formula.

4. *Is there any blood in your baby's stools?*
   If there is, talk to your doctor. This may be a sign of a medical problem, or it may be a sign of food allergy. Blood in a stool may appear black or red. Black colouring can indicate blood from high in the GI tract, whereas red colouring can indicate blood from lower in the GI tract. Blood may even come from what a baby is drinking (damaged nipples can cause some blood to be in the milk). Even small amounts of black or red colouring should be discussed with a doctor, to rule out allergy or other medical issues.

5. *Is your baby congested or do they seem to constantly have a runny nose?*
   If so, your baby may have a cold. If this cold doesn't seem to resolve, and if it is in combination with other digestive problems like mucous in stools or constipation, it may be a sign of allergy. Talk to your doctor.

6. *Does your baby have any skin issues e.g. rashes that seem to flare after feeds, hives, eczema or very dry skin that needs frequent moisturising on a daily basis?*
   In combination with other digestive symptoms like mucous or blood in stools, constipation or diarrhoea this may be a sign of allergy.

7. *Is there a family history of food allergy?*
   Consider both sides of the family and whether there may be allergies which family members had as babies which were outgrown. Also consider whether there are digestive issues which were perhaps never diagnosed as allergy – a family member who feels that dairy or gluten or some other foodstuff just doesn't agree with them, or family members with IBS, Crohn's, or other gut-related conditions.

8. If you feel your baby has a combination of symptoms (digestive, respiratory, skin), talk to your doctor about whether your baby may have an allergy so that you can be referred to a dietitian or allergy clinic. If you are formula feeding you may be prescribed an amino acid (non-dairy formula). If you are breastfeeding, you may also want to talk to an IBCLC or other breastfeeding specialist about breastfeeding a baby with allergy.

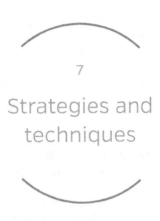

7

Strategies and techniques

This chapter is a set of tips and resources for self-help. It will provide some simple techniques and reference information to help you navigate some of the suggestions in Chapter 6 around weight gain, anxiety and calming techniques.

Switch feeding (breastfeeding only)

Switch feeding maximises intake at the breast by increasing volume at each feed, and reducing the length of the feed. It also increases milk production.

1. Start on the first breast. Watch your baby's swallowing pattern. You will probably notice your baby sucking 3–4 times before each swallow. Within 1–2 minutes you should notice that your baby starts swallowing at each suck, or every other suck. This is a sign that your baby has triggered a milk ejection/letdown and is now getting good milk flow. This will last for 1–2 minutes. Then your baby may go back to 3–4 sucks and a swallow.

2. Swap sides. Repeat Step 1.
3. Swap sides for the second time and allow your baby to feed and then comfort at the breast. If you are not sure when your baby is swallowing or how to identify the milk ejection/letdown, seek breastfeeding support from a qualified breastfeeding counsellor, IBCLC or healthcare professional.

Reducing milk intake at the breast (breastfeeding only)

If your baby has very high weight gain and is comfortable and content there is no need to decrease weight gain. If, however, your baby is gaining much more rapidly than expected and is uncomfortable, gassy and has reflux symptoms then reducing milk intake may help. It's important to do this in a way which still allows your baby to feed frequently and to have all their suckling needs met.

You can reduce your baby's intake by carefully managing how often you switch sides. The more often you switch sides, the more you stimulate milk production. The less often you switch sides, the less you stimulate milk production. If your baby is taking both sides at a feed you may find that offering only one side is all you need to do. If your baby already only takes one side at a feed but feeds quite frequently, then using the same breast for two feeds may be helpful for a few days. Seek breastfeeding support from a qualified breastfeeding counsellor, IBCLC or healthcare professional trained in breastfeeding support in order to determine the right solution for you and how long to maintain it. Having another weight check within 1–2 weeks is helpful to determine how well this is working.

Paced bottle-feeding

Milk flows very differently from the breast and bottle, and very differently depending on how you use a bottle, and it is very easy for babies to overfeed and drink too much milk from a bottle.[1] This may lead to digestive discomfort and reflux-like symptoms. It is estimated that babies may drink an extra 10,000 calories in the first 12 months if they are fed by bottle rather than being fed at the breast. This is important not just for our babies' short-term discomfort, but also for longer-term appetite regulation.[2] Babies who are fed by bottle at 0–3 months are less likely to be responsive to their own signs of fullness at age six. They may have learned to ignore their feelings of fullness.[3]

Research tells us that formula-fed babies drink 49% more milk at one month than breastfed babies, 57% more at three months and 71% more at five months.[4] There may be two reasons for this. The first reason may be the flow rate. When breastfeeding at the breast there are periods of fast milk flow punctuated by periods of slow milk flow. This allows the baby to rest and get ready for the next period of activity and also allows time for the baby to realise that they are getting full. With a bottle the caregiver needs to actively manage the flow rate by changing the angle of the bottle. The second reason may be that we as caregivers have a preconceived idea of how much milk our baby 'should' drink at each feed and we encourage the baby to finish the bottle. We may even put a little extra milk in the bottle 'just in case' and then still encourage our baby to finish the feed.

Paced bottle-feeding is a technique which helps us to give a bottle in a responsive way, to help our baby manage the flow and regulate their appetite. When pacing a feed the baby sits up in our arms, quite vertical, and the bottle is held horizontally (this is different from how we traditionally bottle-feed, with the baby laid down and the bottle tipped up). The bottle is offered to the baby, and only when the baby is sucking in an organised way is the bottle tipped up a little so faster flow begins. After a minute or so (earlier if the baby shows signs of wanting a rest) the bottle is placed horizontally so that flow slows down. The baby is still feeding, but the flow is slow. The baby can stop sucking and rest. Or they can suck slowly, not getting much milk. This is maintained until the baby shows signs of wanting more flow, and then the bottle is tipped up again for just a short time, and this process is repeated throughout the feed. The caregiver watches for signs of being content (fists near the face and body content) or signs of being distressed at flow which is too fast (e.g. splayed hands or furrowed brow). You may also want to use a slower flow teat.

Using a sling/baby carrier

Slings and baby carriers are a great way of increasing contact with your young baby. Babies who are carried a lot tend to be more settled and content and to cry less.[5]

There are multiple different types and designs of slings and carriers, some designed for use from birth and some from a few weeks old, so check the sling/carrier you have chosen is suitable for your baby. If you have a sling library or sling consultant near you they will help you to choose the best option for you. There are also lots of websites with explanatory videos showing how the sling should be used. When using a sling or baby carrier it is very important to follow the TICKS safety guidelines:

- T – *Tight.* You baby should be held close to you with an upright back. If your baby's back slumps away from you this can affect breathing.

- I – *In View At All Times.* When wearing a sling or carrier you should be able to see your baby each time that you glance towards them. Fabric should never close around them so that you have to open it to see your baby.
- C – *Close Enough To Kiss.* Your baby should be high enough on your body that you can kiss them on the head simply by bowing your head towards them.
- K – *Keep Chin Off The Chest.* Make sure that your baby never has their chin resting down on their chest as this can restrict breathing. There should always be a space between their chest and their chin to free the airway.
- S – *Supported Back.* The sling or carrier should provide good back support to prevent the baby's back from slumping in order to protect breathing. When used properly, if you put your hand on your baby's back and apply a little pressure your baby should not move.

Tummy massage

Tummy massage can help with constipation. It is also a very enjoyable activity and provides important sensory input for babies. Babies who are massaged tend to put on weight better and be more settled.[6] There are many different massage techniques and there may be massage classes close to you. There are also many websites and online videos and online classes showing massage techniques. Below I will describe just three techniques which can be helpful for gas and constipation. It is assumed that your baby is healthy and well. It should be enjoyable for your baby. If your baby seems uncomfortable, stop.

Bicycle legs (good for gas)

Lay your baby on their back and gently move their legs in a bicycle motion for a few minutes.

Legs to tummy (good for helping to pass gas)

Lay your baby on their back. Put your hands underneath your baby's knees. Roll your baby's knees up to their tummy. You may hear your baby pass gas as you do this.

I Love You (good for encouraging bowel movement)

This tummy massage follows the pattern of the letters I L U upside-down, hence the name, I Love You. Lay your baby on their back. Use light massage similar to the pressure you might use when applying skin cream. You may want to use a massage oil for babies. Start on the right side of your baby's body (as you look down) and massage downwards from under the rib cage to the top of the leg. That is the 'I' stroke.

Then start on the left side of your baby's body (as you look down) under the rib cage and massage straight across to the right side of the body and then back down the original line to the top of the leg. This is the upside down 'L'. Finally, do the upside-down 'U'. Begin on the left side of your baby's body (as you look down) at the top of the leg. Massage upwards to the rib cage, then across the body, then back down the original line. This is the complete massage. Repeat a few times.

This is a very effective technique. Doing this a few times at each nappy change can encourage regular movement.

Safe bed-sharing/co-sleeping

Young babies should sleep close to a caregiver in order to reduce the risk of SIDS. Some breastfeeding parents may also choose to bed-share, as this makes breastfeeding easier and often helps a baby to sleep better.[7] Bed-sharing is not an option for every family, and should only be done if it can be done safely. Where all the safe sleep guidelines are met, bed-sharing is as safe as a baby sleeping alone. The safe bed-sharing guidelines are as follows:

1. Healthy, full-term baby.
2. Breastfeeding mother and baby.
3. Everyone in the bed should be a non-smoker.
4. No one in the bed should have taken any drugs or medication which might impair their arousal.
5. Baby should be sleeping on their back.
6. Baby shouldn't be dressed in a way which makes them too hot.
7. The sleep surface should be flat (a bed, not a sofa/water bed).

By the time a baby is four months old the research suggests that any sober, non-smoking caregiver can bed-share with a baby, not just a breastfeeding mother.

If you are formula-feeding you may want to consider something like a co-sleeper cot/crib which allows your baby to be close to you, but on a separate sleep surface. For further evidence-based information on safe sleep for your baby, however they are fed, a good resource is the Baby Sleep Information Source based at Durham University. (www.basisonline.org.uk)

> *'I think it's ingrained in us that if our baby cries then it's reflux or wind. I was so worried about this I fell asleep in unsafe positions sitting up to keep her head elevated, until I lay down and fell asleep with her on the breast and she barely made a peep. My baby did cry out often but all*

she seemed to want was me. It fixed everything when I gave her just that.' Emma

Reducing anxiety and worry

Having an unsettled baby is very worrying. If your baby is not sleeping or feeding as you expected, this is worrying. If your baby is vomiting a lot and not gaining weight, this is worrying. If your baby is crying most of the day, it is very distressing. These daily worries cause us to feel stressed and anxious. Our babies sense this stress response. They don't know why we are worried, but they get the message that we don't feel safe right now. This causes our babies to become stressed too. This impairs digestion and often means that babies do not feed or sleep well. This makes us more worried and causes a vicious cycle of anxiety.

Reducing the stress response in your body will help your baby to relax more, and this in turn will help your baby's digestion, feeding and sleep. Listening to mindfulness apps or relaxation tracks during the day can help to reduce the nervous system arousal in your body and reduce muscle tension. When holding or feeding your baby you can use your own relaxation as a strategy to help your baby relax. If your baby is unsettled, try moving or swaying, and use breath techniques to reduce stress in your body. One of the most effective methods is to make your out-breath a little longer than your in-breath. Try breathing in for a count of four, then out for a count of seven. Repeating this a few times can be very effective at calming you both.

Learning about how my anxiety affects my baby was a game changer for me. I made a conscious decision to be "present" during feeds and shut out the things I felt I should hurry up to get to, like washing. The difference it

made to us as a dyad was incredible, and I wouldn't have believed if I hadn't experienced it. Claire

Singing naturally produces a rhythm of short in-breaths and longer out-breaths, which may be one of the reasons that singing helps to settle babies. So even if you don't think you are a good singer, try singing and moving with your baby.

If you are worried for large parts of the day every day, or you seem to be spending a lot of time researching information on reflux or unsettled babies then consider reaching out for some expert help. If you have already had help resolving symptoms as much as possible but still find yourself very anxious, CBT (cognitive behavioural therapy) can be a very helpful intervention. We do know that parental stress and anxiety is linked with the diagnosis of reflux in babies.[8]

Tummy time

Tummy time is important for developing core strength and meeting milestones like sitting. We know that reflux reduces significantly once a baby is able to sit upright. Tummy time is also important for coordination and optimal nervous system development and this helps with a baby's ability to transition between states and to calm and soothe.

The research suggests that a baby should spend 90 minutes a day in tummy time. Many parents say that their baby doesn't like tummy time and this is why they don't spend much time doing it. There can be a few reasons why babies don't like tummy time, and it is easy to change the way we do it to help babies to enjoy it more.

1. The way they are placed into tummy time can be unsettling. How they are set down can produce very different sensations. Lifting a baby, flipping them over and

setting them on the floor is a massive sensory experience. In many ways it may feel like a rollercoaster ride for a baby. Instead, try laying your baby on their back, spend a short time chatting and playing with them and when they are settled, try rolling them on to their tummy.

2. Babies need to see us. Babies feel safe when we are with them and making them feel safe. If they are on their tummies on the floor and we are standing nearby or sitting a few feet away, they cannot see our eyes. Babies can start to get dysregulated quickly without us. Try getting down on the floor with your baby, looking into their eyes and playing with them there.

3. Young babies may only want to stay in tummy time for a short period, but if you do short periods many times throughout the day it can add up to quite a lot of time, and over a few weeks each individual time will get longer. Try adding in a little tummy time at each nappy change, or letting your baby nap on your chest on their tummy to build up the time.

Investigating food allergy

If you are seeing symptoms in multiple body systems (e.g. mucous/blood in stools, combined with skin rashes, congestion in the nose/runny nose) alongside feeding problems then you may want to investigate food allergy. You should always discuss allergy symptoms with your doctor.

The most common food allergy in babies is cow's milk protein allergy. This isn't surprising given that milk is babies' sole food stuff for around six months, and many babies are fed using infant formula (created from cow's milk). Many babies who react to cow's milk protein also react to soy protein. The next most common allergen is egg, but babies can react to many different types of food just as adults do. I have worked with babies with confirmed allergies to gluten, coconut oil, oats, bananas and sesame, among other things. I have also worked with babies who didn't have confirmed allergy, nor GORD, but who vomited more when the breastfeeding mother ate a particular food.

Identifying a food allergen can be tricky. There are two main types of food allergy: IgE allergies and non-IgE allergies. IgE allergies are so called because the immune reaction involves a particular type of antibody, called IgE. IgE reactions tend to appear very shortly after eating the food. It may be immediate, or within the next couple of hours. The reactions are often swelling or rashes. A non-IgE allergy involves different parts of the immune system and the symptoms are much more delayed, usually appearing several hours to a couple of days after eating the allergen. The symptoms are generally more chronic, such as eczema, constipation and irritability, for example. IgE allergies can be identified with skin-prick tests, but there is no reliable test for non-IgE allergies. The gold standard to test for a non-IgE allergy is to eliminate a food for a trial period of around two weeks to see if the symptoms resolve. If the symptoms resolve the food is reintroduced. If symptoms return that is a positive test.

If you are formula-feeding and your baby is not yet having solid foods, elimination is fairly simple as you can remove the dairy formula and swap to an amino-acid formula for a trial. If you find your baby is allergic to dairy you may even consider relactation and beginning to breastfeed (at least for some feeds).

If you are breastfeeding, it can be more difficult to identify a food allergen, but while you are figuring it out your baby continues to get breastmilk packed with anti-inflammatories and factors which promote gut health. Examining your family history can be a helpful first step. If you have family members who react to dairy, then that increases the risk that dairy is the allergen for your baby. If you have family members who are coeliac and you are eating a lot of bread, that may be an indicator that the amount of bread you are eating is the issue.

A food diary can be very helpful. With a food diary, you write down every food or drink that you consume and note how your baby's temperament was that day along with any symptoms that you noticed. It's important to look at the diary over the course of a week, as symptoms from a food may appear the day after eating it. There are also apps and books which will help you with this process. A book which I highly recommend to help you understand food allergy in babies and how to identify food allergens is *Crying Babies & Food* by Maureen Minchin.[9]

If you find that you are eliminating more and more foods and your diet is getting more and more restricted without resolving your baby's symptoms, reach out for help from a professional. It is very easy for breastfeeding mums to make their diet too restricted and for this to create further problems with feeding.

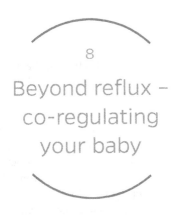

8

Beyond reflux – co-regulating your baby

'Nothing an infant can or cannot do makes sense, except in light of the mother's body.' Nils Bergman[1]

What if I told you that the reason there is such a difference in what you expected of your baby (three-hourly feeds, ability to sleep alone, ability to be laid down) and the reality (frequent cueing for feeds, wanting to be held and to sleep on you) is because you have been fed inaccurate expectations throughout your life?

What if I told you that Western society's understanding of babies and what babies need is flawed?

What if I told you that your baby needs your body intensely, just so their body works properly?

Our babies need a lot of care. In order to understand how much, I need you to suspend all your current beliefs about babies and about parents. Put everything that society has told you on hold, and think about our babies as you would look at another species.

The baby primate

The first thing to understand is that our babies are born with very immature brains, and that immaturity means that our babies are not capable of doing very much to keep themselves safe and alive. Other mammals that we are used to seeing on farms (cows, horses, sheep, goats, pigs) have babies who are able to get to their feet very quickly and follow their mother around. They can flee from predators. They can find their way to their mother if they are separated and can initiate feeding.

In stark contrast a primate baby, such as a chimp or gorilla baby, is able to cling to their mother and spends most of their time on the mother's body. They stay attached to their mother's front for 3–6 months, then move to their mother's back. At the age of around two they will start to climb down from their mother, venturing up to 16ft away before returning to their mother's back. They only start sleeping on their own at around 4–5 years of age.

That's a long time for an infant chimp to need to be attached to their mother, and a baby chimp is actually more mature than a baby human. At birth, an ape's brain is about 50% the size of an adult ape brain. A human baby at birth, however, has a brain which is only about 25% of its adult brain mass. Our babies cannot venture away from us and return. They can't get away from danger. They can't make their way to us if they need to feed or have some other need met. They can't even cling to us. This means they are entirely dependent upon us to care for them. Their biological expectation is that we will behave much like the chimp mother. This means that babies need an awful lot of time, attention and work – perhaps much more than you have been led to expect.

Why would evolution/nature design our babies to be so helpless and to need so much energy and labour from the parent? The answer lies in our pelvis. If we were to let our baby's brain grow to 50% of their adult size they would have a much larger head at birth. Since we birth that head through our pelvis that would mean we would need to have a much larger pelvis. A larger pelvis is heavy – too heavy for walking upright. An ape can pass a much larger head through its heavy pelvis because they walk on four limbs, but an animal that walks on two legs has to have a much smaller and lighter pelvis, and therefore can only give birth to a baby with a smaller brain. At some stage in the past we as a species made an unconscious evolutionary decision about walking upright. As an evolutionary trade-off for the advantage of being bipedal, our baby's gestation changed. Rather than having a gestation completely inside the womb (like a calf for example) we created a situation where we split a baby's gestation into two parts. Part of it inside the womb, and part of it outside the womb but in our arms. A baby is much like a kangaroo joey. A joey is born, makes its way to the pouch, climbs inside, drinks milk and completes its gestation. Our human babies are born, are placed in our arms, feed at the breast and complete gestation there. Our arms are our pouch.

Those small, immature brains aren't very good at keeping the body systems stable. As mature adults we can keep our heart rates regular, we can bring our breathing under voluntary control, we manage our temperature. We can look out for threats. We can recognise our emotions (usually) and we have learned to manage our stress and our emotional responses to some degree. Our babies cannot do any of these things well. They aren't even very good at the basic things, like stable regular breathing, heart rate or temperature unless they are on an adult body.[2] You may even have noticed that if lying alone sometimes your baby might seem to stop breathing for a brief moment. Babies cannot regulate these systems themselves, but they can 'borrow' our adult regulation when held against an adult body. That adult keeps the baby's body systems regulated. The adult heart rate regulates the baby's heart rate, the stable adult breathing regulates the baby's breathing and the adult temperature regulates the baby's temperature. Babies literally need our bodies. They need their body to be against ours. This is co-regulation, a state where the adult is required to regulate the infant's body. Research tells us that: *'The science behind reproductive biology is that all of a mother's body sensations help control all of the different parts of the physiology of the baby.'* [3]

'I was always told a newborn baby sleeps all of the time and only wakes to feed. They should be laid in their cot/ pram. How are we given such false ideas?' Emma

Society may tell us that we should be able to put our babies down, and that they should be able to sleep alone, but neuroscience tells us that when babies are separated from us, even by a couple of feet, their bodies become dysregulated. They become stressed. They move into a fight or flight state, and once they do that, they release stress hormones. When releasing stress hormones they are not releasing growth hormone. Once they are picked up again, they become regulated, they calm and they begin releasing growth hormone again. This is why babies who are massaged (involving safe and relaxing touch) grow faster than babies who receive less touch.

This means it is completely normal for a young baby to want to be in your arms almost all the time. Their body expects to be in your arms almost all the time. In order to feel safe, secure and to be growing optimally, they need to be attached to a mature adult nervous system in order to regulate their own. This period of exterogestation is the fourth trimester, completing the pregnancy. In the womb the baby's body has developed enough to survive without the womb, placenta and amniotic fluid, but now they need the proximity of a regulating nervous system. It won't always be this way, but it is at the start.

It is no surprise to me that the majority of babies who are treated for or labelled as having reflux/GORD are within the first few weeks of life. They are within the fourth trimester period and attempts to parent them like an older baby lead to dysregulation and reflux-like symptoms. There is a mismatch between our expectations for basic care around feeding, sleeping, carrying and our baby's fourth trimester needs.

Feeding and digestion

As adults, we are very aware of the link between our stress levels and our digestion. We say we have butterflies in our tummy when we are nervous. We know the effect fear has on our bowels, and how it causes feelings of nausea. Babies feel stress if dysregulated, and they become dysregulated quickly when out of the arms of an adult caregiver. Is it any surprise, then, that babies who are not in arms for much of the day might have problems with digestion: gas, colic, reflux symptoms?

Then there is normal feeding frequency to consider. A newborn is designed to feed frequently. At birth a newborn's stomach has a capacity of about 30ml. When milk comes in, the volume of milk in one letdown/milk ejection is also around 30ml. This means that a baby is likely designed to feed very small amounts very frequently. At one week old, for example, that could mean that a baby feeds 18 times a day.

That's approximately every 90 mins, or there may be hourly clustering of feeds, and then a longer gap for sleep. In Western society that might seem impossible, but it is, and has been, how babies are cared for in other societies. A 1969 and 1971 study observing the !Kung San peoples in Botswana found that babies often fed four times per hour.[4] These were short feeds, taking only a few minutes. Babies were carried 80% of the time and cried only 10–20% of the time that babies in London cry.

In my experience there is a middle ground. If babies are carried for most of the day, fed and then held in a sling they usually don't feed more than once an hour, and they are also very settled.

Sharing sleep or solitary sleep

How many times have you found that your baby fed to sleep, or drifted peacefully asleep in your arms, but within a few minutes of being laid down in a cot, they woke? I dare say all parents have found this. We search for solutions. We try warming the cot so the baby will not notice the shift to a cold surface. We try swaddling so that the baby still feels like they are in arms. We try womb sounds or white noise to remind them of the womb. We try shushing, or rocking, but none of these things will fool your baby into thinking they are still in your arms, because they are no longer being regulated. A warm surface can't regulate their heart rate or their brainwaves. Neither can a swaddle, or shushing. In chapters 4 and 5 we talked briefly about sleep cycles. Passing through entire sleep cycles (light sleep to deep sleep, then back up through light sleep, dreams, brief awakening) is part of the process of memory formation. Each step in the cycle is required to form memories in the brain. The cycling process is how we wire connections in this little immature brain and how we grow and mature it. Sleep cycling happens when a baby is held in arms, or sleeping against a body, but it is disrupted when a baby is out of arms. The dysregulated baby does not sleep cycle.

'The swaddled and separated baby lies still with its eyes closed, and is believed to be sleeping. A study on autonomic activation,[6] showed that quiet sleep was reduced by 86% in separated babies and their sleep cycling was almost abolished.' Nils Bergman, 2014 [2]

Babies don't wake when we put them down because the cot is too cold. They wake because the adult body is no longer regulating and stabilising their body, and so their body doesn't work properly.

That might leave you wondering how you can possibly get any sleep. Maybe you can let your baby nap in a sling during the day, but what can you do at night? Part of the reason you are querying reflux may be because you need to get more sleep at night, and feel like your baby should be sleeping longer.

Babies need us at night for a long time. Waking and needing our help to regulate, to calm the nervous system and drift back to sleep is needed for a long time. In general babies are not sleeping long stretches until they are around a year old. In fact at 12 months 27% of babies are not regularly sleeping an eight-hour stretch (what we as adults consider to be normal for us).[7] That's over a quarter of all babies. Even those babies will be waking some nights for help. Chimp babies sleep alone (meaning they can manage their own needs) at around 4–5 years, and the development of the skill of self-management at night is probably not on much of a different timeline for many human babies.

So how do we cope? Many of us find that we get more sleep by sleeping close to our babies. If breastfeeding, and we can do so safely, we may choose to bed-share. It may surprise you to know that half of parents in the UK bedshare in the first three months, but many don't talk about it.[8] In Japan, where co-sleeping and breastfeeding is the cultural norm, rates of SIDS are the lowest in the world.[9] Sleeping with our babies gives us more sleep and better quality sleep. 84% of bed-sharing mothers report 'good' or 'enough' sleep vs only 64% of solitary sleeping mothers. We also know that the average duration of awakenings is shorter for bed-sharing mothers.[10]

Often when we are struggling with sleep it's because we are trying to make our baby fit our adult sleep schedule... but their brain just isn't developed enough to do it. We are fighting biology. Fighting biology usually ends in failure and then a sense of self-blame and defeat because we can't change the situation. What can help is trying to adapt to the baby. Sleep like your baby sleeps until your baby is mature enough to sleep like you. That means forgetting about the housework, and giving yourself permission to lie down during the day and take a nap. Re-invigorate the siesta. Ask for help from friends or family to look after your baby so that you can get some sleep.

Co-regulation <–> dysregulation

Our bodies are regulated when we feel safe. A sense of safety is the key to optimal health and growth. You may have learned that when we are unsafe/under threat we move into a fight or flight state. The reality is slightly more complex. As mammals, we have a social component to our nervous system. Our physiology and behaviours are directly impacted by our social circumstances, our connection to other people, our environment and our perception of all of these factors. This is true of adults, just as it is true of babies.

The social nervous system has a more nuanced response to threat than just fight or flight.[11]

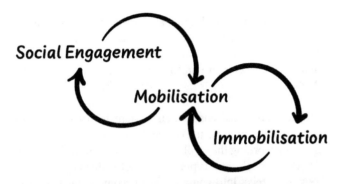

When we are faced with a threat, firstly mammals try to resolve the problem socially. If you are out at an event and a fire alarm sounds, it's unlikely that you will run out instantly (flight) or that you will start searching for the fire in order to tackle it (fight). It's likely that you will engage with other humans nearby. You might ask them, 'Is that the fire alarm? Do you think it is real, or a test? Do you think we should leave?' We look for some kind of common consensus about the threat level. We socially engage. If we are told, 'It's a test. It was scheduled for this time', the threat has been eliminated and we stay in social engagement. We are safe. We relax. If, however we are told, 'It's real, we need to evacuate,' we will move into the next level of our threat system. This is 'fight or flight'. We release adrenaline and cortisol. We increase blood flow to our muscles. We increase our heart rate and our breathing rate. We prepare to move, to mobilise. This is when we might pick up our things and flee, or try to tackle/fight the problem. If we resolve the problem we can then move back into social engagement and a sense of safety. If we do not resolve the problem we move into our final threat coping system – immobilisation. This is 'freeze'. If you have ever seen an animal under threat playing dead, this is the freeze system at work.

How might this work in a baby? What do I mean when I talk about dysregulation? Let's take a baby who is lying alone. Perhaps they have been out of arms for a little while and so their body systems are starting to become less organised. Maybe their breathing is less regular. Maybe their brainwaves become altered. This is a threat to a young baby. They first activate their social engagement system to try to get your attention. They might grunt or search for you with their eyes. If this is not working they will likely become more verbal. If you pick up your baby at this point, and soothe them against your body, they relax into you and they become regulated. They may even make eye contact to seal that social engagement. They feel safe again. All is right with their world.

If the baby's needs are not met immediately, they become more dysregulated and feel more threat, and they move into the mobilisation system. This mobilisation will be seen as increased movements in the arms and legs. Then they will start to cry loudly. Their limbs will start to flail. They are desperate to get your attention. This crying causes reduced oxygen, increased blood pressure in the brain, increased heart rate and increased blood pressure. This puts the body at even greater threat. If you pick up your baby at this point and soothe them against your body the threat disappears. It may take a few minutes longer but they relax into you as they become regulated. All is right with their world.

If the baby's needs are still not met at the mobilisation stage, they move into the final threat state – immobilisation. This is what happens when a crying baby suddenly quietens down and seems to fall asleep. It looks like they are peacefully asleep, but they have actually entered a state of immobilisation in which they are not sleep cycling.

This description shouldn't make you feel like all crying will be harmful to your baby. Crying is part of being a baby. The stress comes from not being responded to. A baby who is crying in arms, while being tended to and loved, is in a very different stress state to a baby who is crying alone. Babies will cry. All babies will cry. All babies will have an increase in crying in the weeks following birth, easing off by around 12 weeks (the end of the fourth trimester). Carrying your baby and holding them as much as possible will reduce the crying dramatically, but some crying is very normal. The study of the !Kung San babies found that even these babies had an increase in crying over the first three months. A Danish community survey found that babies had a peak of crying at around three weeks.[12] The duration of crying was lower than the average in other industrialised countries and this was thought to be due to the Danish mothers' prompt responses to their babies, but even in the Danish group some babies cried a lot.

Another study looking at babies in London and Denmark found that although crying and fussing at 10 days and five weeks was less in the group who were held for longer, episodes of intense inconsolable crying were equally common across groups.[13] Sometimes babies cry, and it doesn't mean that they are in pain. If we don't expect crying we can easily think that something is wrong, and reach for a label like reflux.

Sometimes crying is developmental. Sometimes we don't know what is happening, but we know that crying increases around the same timeframes for most babies, so it is likely that something neurobiological is happening. It's stressful as a parent to listen to crying. The crying is part of a threat system, and it triggers our own threat system. It is anxiety-producing – but that doesn't always mean that there is something wrong and that our baby is in pain.

Sometimes crying is excessive. Around 5% of babies follow Wessel's 'rule of 3s' for colic (crying for three hours a day, at least three days a week, for at least three weeks).[14] A very interesting new theory of colic is that it is a glitch in the breathing system.[15] As adults we have two breathing modes. We have our automatic breathing system, which takes care of our breathing when we aren't thinking about it. We also have our voluntary breathing system which we use for speech. When we talk we have to carefully control our breath so that we can make words, sentences and have spaces between sounds. We swap seamlessly between the two systems.

Babies, in contrast, only have their reflex breathing system active at birth. This is why crying in a young baby is quite full on and sustained, compared to an older baby who might whimper or whine and has different vocal qualities to their cries. Babies need to develop voluntary breath control in order to vocalise (speech breathing). James McKenna theorises that colic is a glitch in the developing system in which a baby tries to switch from reflex breathing to speech breathing as they start to cry, but the glitch means that both systems activate at once. The baby is now crying and is unable to stop. The crying can be prolonged until one system deactivates. This is a very interesting theory and colic crying fits neatly with speech breathing development. The important takeaway is that crying can often be due to something developmental that we don't understand, and it doesn't mean a baby is in pain. If we have tried our best to meet all of our baby's needs and they are still crying, perhaps it is one of these developmental stages and we have to ride it out.

Thriving in the fourth trimester

'The moment a child is born, the mother is also born. She never existed before. The woman existed, but the mother, never. A mother is something absolutely new.' Osho

A baby arriving is a shock to the system of life that we have created around us. It disrupts our sense of control in our lives, our ability to get adequate sleep, our ability to do the things we want to do when we want to do them. It disrupts our sense of who we are and how we and our partners, families and friends interact and function together.

We have no idea when our baby is going to want to feed, or how long that feed might last. We have no idea when the next sleep is coming, or how long it might be. Our baby intensely needs to be held, to be fed, to comfort suck, to be regulated and soothed and given constant care. It's exhausting. Many of us expect this with a newborn, but as the days turn into weeks and we are still finding the intensity of baby care difficult and the lack of sleep hard to cope with, we start to long for some kind of structure, some sense of control of our lives again. To add to this we often start getting questions from family and friends about whether our little one is in a routine, whether they are sleeping well for us and so on. All of this is a perfect recipe for anxiety and stress and in response to that an unsettled baby. When we don't know when we will be able to eat or sleep, our own bodies feel under threat.

When we feel out of control we don't feel competent. We often want to regain some control, and when we look around for a way to regain that control that we are presented with marketing about problems that can be solved. We are sold sleep programmes, feeding programmes, baby care programmes, and medical conditions with pharmaceutical solutions.

The vast majority of these programmes and solutions don't take into account the development in the fourth trimester, and a baby's intense physiological needs. They also ignore the fact that we can't actually control other people. We can't control when our baby will drift from a deep sleep into a light sleep and wake any more than we can control when our neighbour wakes or leaves the house. We can't control how long a feed will take, or how our baby will manage that feed. We can't control other people. We can only control ourselves, and sometimes we even struggle with that. Trying to change our young baby's behaviour to make it more structured is just another fight against biology. Babies' needs do get less intense as they mature, but time is the only solution to that.

So how can we shift from just surviving through the fourth trimester to thriving through the fourth trimester? These are some steps that might help:

1. Remember that your baby is not trying to manipulate you if they are crying to be picked up and carried again. They really do need you. Their body just doesn't work properly without you. The neuroscience is really clear – babies have the best developmental outcomes if they are responded to promptly. You are doing the best for your baby by carrying them.

2. You don't have to respond to advice from others. People may tell you what your baby should or shouldn't be doing, but that doesn't mean they are correct. You are the expert on your baby. You know what makes your baby happiest.

3. Know that it's okay to feel overwhelmed. Young babies need our bodies to regulate them and that puts a big demand on us. Sometimes it's just too much for one or two people. It's okay to ask for help. It doesn't mean that we are failing as parents. In fact it shows that we are being

responsive to both our baby's and our own needs. Robin Grille (a neurosocial psychologist) has stated that for most of human history (i.e. pre-history) human babies were surrounded by at least four adults.[16] It's much easier for four adults to meet the needs of one baby. We can't expect to do it all ourselves. It really does take a village to raise a child.

4. Take care of your mental health. Having a new baby makes us more anxious. Some anxiety is completely normal, and is likely part of the bonding and attachment process, but if we are not looking after our own needs as well, it is easy for that anxiety to become a problem. Remember that you can only regulate another person if you are well regulated yourself. If we are very anxious and our anxious body is trying to regulate our baby, our baby becomes more unsettled and this can create a vicious cycle of anxiety and unsettled behaviour. Look at your day and your week and ensure that you have some time to do things that you enjoy. Those might be with your baby, or without them. It might be a bath or a walk or reading, drawing, meeting friends. It doesn't matter what it is, as long as you are getting some pleasure and relaxation from it. Using relaxation or mindfulness apps can also help to relax your nervous system, which helps you to calm your baby too.

5. Parenting is about a relationship – not getting it 'right' all the time. Parenting is hard and exhausting because we are complex animals with large social and intelligent brains. Helping our babies become those complex animals with large social and intelligent brains requires us to invest a lot of our resources into our babies. It is challenging and we will make mistakes. We won't always get our responsive parenting right. We will make mistakes. We will do things that are not so loving and responsive at times. That's okay!

It's important to know it's okay. Research tells us that in healthy attached relationships parents are only perfectly in tune with their baby about one third of the time. For another third they are not tuned in well to them, and for the final third they are trying to repair and get back in tune.[17] We don't have to be perfect. We can't be perfect. That means it's also okay if your family or the support network you draw on for help doesn't do things exactly the same way that you do. We can't control other relationships, just our own. It's okay for them to do things differently when they care for your baby and for you to do them your way when you do.

The fourth trimester is intense but can also be wonderful. There will never be another time when your baby needs you so intensely, and you are so close that you share a nervous system. If you can reframe the constant need for you from something negative to something positive it can be beautiful. It is hard to find something more fulfilling than your baby melting into your body and the wave of love that you both feel. It's okay to hold your baby a lot. It's creating a loving, trusting relationship with your baby. It's good to hold your baby. Responding as best we can, as much as we can, will help our baby grow and thrive, as well as making for a less anxious, calmer household. It floods you both with oxytocin, and that is not a bad habit. More oxytocin creates a brain oriented towards love. A brain oriented towards love, that is well regulated as a baby and growing child, is more resilient and better able to deal with stress as an adult. You are shaping the future for your baby. Could anything be more important or wonderful?

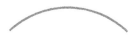

Acknowledgements

I'd like to thank those who played a role in bringing this book to life, which was several years in the writing. Thank you to my parents, who instilled in me the determination and drive. Thank you to my husband for his support when I gave up a corporate career to mother our children and help other mothers. Thank you to all those mothers I have worked with for allowing me into their lives and trusting me to be part of their experience. More than anyone, however, I say thank you to my two children, Will and Lucas, who turned my life upside down, introduced me to the joy of mothering through breastfeeding, and taught me about reflux, the social nervous system and the wonders of oxytocin. You are both amazing and I am so proud of you.

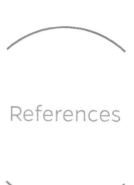

References

Chapter 1: Understanding reflux

1. Ravinder K. Mittal, M.D., Raj K. Goyal, M.D. (2006) Sphincter mechanisms at the lower end of the esophagus. *GI Motility online* (2006) doi:10.1038/gimo14
2. Cavell B. Gastric emptying in infants fed human milk or infant formula. *Acta Paediatr Scand.* 1981;70(5):639-641.
3. Ana Ruigómez, Mari-Ann Wallander, Per Lundborg, Saga Johansson & Luis A. Garcia Rodriguez (2010) Gastroesophageal reflux disease in children and adolescents in primary care. *Scandinavian Journal of Gastroenterology,* 45:2, 139-146, DOI: 10.3109/00365520903428606
4. Mitchell DJ, McClure BG, Tubman TRJ Simultaneous monitoring of gastric and oesophageal pH reveals limitations of conventional oesophageal pH monitoring in milk fed infants. *Archives of Disease in Childhood* 2001;84:273-276.
5. Ana Ruigómez, Mari-Ann Wallander, Per Lundborg, Saga Johansson & Luis A. Garcia Rodriguez (2010) Gastroesophageal reflux disease in children and adolescents in primary care. *Scandinavian Journal of Gastroenterology,* 45:2, 139-146, DOI: 10.3109/00365520903428606
6. Orenstein SR, Hassall E, Furmaga-Jablonska W, Atkinson S, Raanan M. Multicenter, double-blind, randomized, placebo-controlled trial assessing the efficacy and safety of proton pump inhibitor lansoprazole in infants with symptoms of gastroesophageal reflux disease. *J Pediatr.* 2009;154(4):514-520.e4.

7. Moore, David & Tao, Billy & Lines, David & Hirte, Craig & Heddle, Margaret & Davidson, Geoffrey. (2003). Double-blind placebo-controlled trial of omeprazole in irritable infants with gastroesophageal reflux. *The Journal of Pediatrics*. 143. 219-23. 10.1067/S0022-3476(03)00207-5.

8. Hassall E. Over-prescription of acid-suppressing medications in infants: how it came about, why it's wrong, and what to do about it. *J Pediatr*. 2012;160(2):193-198.

9. Blank ML, Parkin L. National Study of Off-label Proton Pump Inhibitor Use Among New Zealand Infants in the First Year of Life (2005-2012). *J Pediatr Gastroenterol Nutr*. 2017;65(2):179-184. doi:10.1097/MPG.0000000000001596

Chapter 2: The role of stomach acid

1. Agunod, M., Yamaguchi, N., Lopez, R. et al. Correlative study of hydrochloric acid, pepsin, and intrinsic factor secretion in newborns and infants. *Digest Dis Sci* 14, 400–414 (1969). https://doi.org/10.1007/BF02239360

2. Zhu H, Hart CA, Sales D, Roberts NB. Bacterial killing in gastric juice-effect of pH and pepsin on Escherichia coli and Helicobacter pylori. *J Med Microbiol*. 2006;55(Pt 9):1265-1270. doi:10.1099/jmm.0.46611-0

3. Bergman NJ. Neonatal stomach volume and physiology suggest feeding at 1-h intervals. *Acta Paediatr*. 2013;102(8):773-777. doi:10.1111/apa.12291

4. Tobey NA, Hosseini SS, Caymaz-Bor C, Wyatt HR, Orlando GS, Orlando RC. The role of pepsin in acid injury to esophageal epithelium. *Am J Gastroenterol*. 2001;96(11):3062-3070. doi:10.1111/j.1572-0241.2001.05260.x

5. Orlando, Roy C. The integrity of the esophageal mucosa. Balance between offensive and defensive mechanisms. Best practice & research. *Clinical Gastroenterology* vol. 24,6 (2010): 873-82. doi:10.1016/j.bpg.2010.08.008

6. Barlow WJ, Orlando RC. The pathogenesis of heartburn in nonerosive reflux disease: a unifying hypothesis. *Gastroenterology*. 2005;128(3):771-778. doi:10.1053/j.gastro.2004.08.014

7. Weijenborg PW, Smout AJ, Verseijden C, et al. Hypersensitivity to acid is associated with impaired esophageal mucosal integrity in patients with gastroesophageal reflux disease with and without esophagitis. *Am J Physiol Gastrointest Liver Physiol*. 2014;307(3):G323-G329. doi:10.1152/ajpgi.00345.2013

8. Weidinger S, O'Sullivan M, Illig T, et al. Filaggrin mutations, atopic eczema, hay fever, and asthma in children. *J Allergy Clin Immunol*. 2008;121(5):1203-1209.e1. doi:10.1016/j.jaci.2008.02.014

9. Esparza-Gordillo J, Matanovic A, Marenholz I, et al. Maternal filaggrin mutations increase the risk of atopic dermatitis in children: an effect independent of mutation inheritance. *PLoS Genet.* 2015;11(3):e1005076. Published 2015 Mar 10. doi:10.1371/journal.pgen.1005076

10. Venkataraman D, Soto-Ramírez N, Kurukulaaratchy RJ, et al. Filaggrin loss-of-function mutations are associated with food allergy in childhood and adolescence. *J Allergy Clin Immunol.* 2014;134(4):876-882.e4. doi:10.1016/j.jaci.2014.07.033

11. Gonzalez Ballesteros, Luisa F et al. Unexpected widespread hypophosphatemia and bone disease associated with elemental formula use in infants and children. *Bone* vol. 97 (2017): 287-292. doi:10.1016/j.bone.2017.02.003

Chapter 3: Reflux treatments and side-effects

1. NICE Guidance on GORD in children. https://www.nice.org.uk/media/default/about/what-we-do/nice-guidance/gord-in-children-full-guideline-draft.pdf

2. Huang RC, Forbes DA, Davies MW. Feed thickener for newborn infants with gastro-oesophageal reflux. *Cochrane Database Syst Rev.* 2002;(3):CD003211. doi:10.1002/14651858.CD003211

3. https://infantmilkinfo.org/wp-content/uploads/2020/03/Anti-Reflux_Infant-Milk_March2020.pdf

4. Carroll AE, Garrison MM, Christakis DA. A Systematic Review of Nonpharmacological and Nonsurgical Therapies for Gastroesophageal Reflux in Infants. *Arch Pediatr Adolesc Med.* 2002;156(2):109–113. doi:10.1001/archpedi.156.2.109

5. Bosscher, Douwina & Caillie-Bertrand, Micheline & Deelstra, Hendrik. (2001). Effect of thickening agents, based on soluble dietary fiber, on the availability of calcium, iron, and zinc from infant formulas. *Nutrition* 17. 614-8. 10.1016/S0899-9007(01)00541-X.

6. Mandel KG, Daggy BP, Brodie DA, Jacoby HI. Alginate-raft formulations in the treatment of heartburn and acid reflux. *Aliment Pharmacol Ther.* 2000;14(6):669-690. doi:10.1046/j.1365-2036.2000.00759.x

7. AS Sandberg, H Andersson, I Bosœus, NG Carlsson, K Hasselblad, M Härröd. Alginate, small bowel sterol excretion, and absorption of nutrients in ileostomy subjects. *The American Journal of Clinical Nutrition*, Volume 60, Issue 5, November 1994, Pages 751–756, https://doi.org/10.1093/ajcn/60.5.751

8. Georg Jensen M, Kristensen M, Astrup A. Effect of alginate supplementation on weight loss in obese subjects completing a 12-wk energy-restricted diet: a randomized controlled trial. *Am J Clin Nutr.* 2012;96(1):5-13. doi:10.3945/ajcn.111.025312

9. El Khoury, D., Goff, H., Berengut, S. et al. Effect of sodium alginate addition to chocolate milk on glycemia, insulin, appetite and food intake in healthy adult men. *Eur J Clin Nutr* 68, 613–618 (2014). https://doi.org/10.1038/ejcn.2014.53

10. Paxman JR, Richardson JC, Dettmar PW, Corfe BM. Daily ingestion of alginate reduces energy intake in free-living subjects. *Appetite.* 2008;51(3):713-719. doi:10.1016/j.appet.2008.06.013

11. Hoad CL, Rayment P, Spiller RC, et al. In vivo imaging of intragastric gelation and its effect on satiety in humans. *J Nutr.* 2004;134(9):2293-2300. doi:10.1093/jn/134.9.2293

12. Dr Jack Newman & Theresa Pitman. *Dr Jack Newman's Guide to Breast-feeding*, revised edition. Pinter & Martin 2014

13. van der Pol RJ, Smits MJ, van Wijk MP, Omari TI, Tabbers MM, Benninga MA. Efficacy of proton-pump inhibitors in children with gastroesophageal reflux disease: a systematic review. *Pediatrics.* 2011;127(5):925-935. doi:10.1542/peds.2010-2719

14. Susan R. Orenstein, Eric Hassall, Wanda Furmaga-Jablonska, Stuart Atkinson, Marsha Raanan. Multicenter, Double-Blind, Randomized, Placebo-Controlled Trial Assessing the Efficacy and Safety of Proton Pump Inhibitor Lansoprazole in Infants with Symptoms of Gastroesophageal Reflux Disease. *The Journal of Pediatrics*, Volume 154, Issue 4, 2009, Pages 514-520.e4, ISSN 0022-3476, doi.org/10.1016/j.jpeds.2008.09.054.

15. Moore, David & Tao, Billy & Lines, David & Hirte, Craig & Heddle, Margaret & Davidson, Geoffrey. (2003). Double-blind placebo-controlled trial of omeprazole in irritable infants with gastroesophageal reflux. *The Journal of Pediatrics.* 143. 219-23. 10.1067/S0022-3476(03)00207-5

16. https://www.medicines.org.uk/emc/files/pil.2326.pdf

17. https://www.medicines.org.uk/emc/PIL.3487.latest.pdf

18. https://www.medicines.org.uk/emcmobile/PIL.26193.latest.pdf

19. Ward, Robert M, and Gregory L Kearns. Proton pump inhibitors in pediatrics : mechanism of action, pharmacokinetics, pharmacogenetics, and pharmacodynamics. *Paediatric Drugs* vol. 15,2 (2013): 119-31. doi:10.1007/s40272-013-0012-x

20. Heidelbaugh, Joel J. Proton pump inhibitors and risk of vitamin and mineral deficiency: evidence and clinical implications. *Therapeutic Advances in Drug Safety* vol. 4,3 (2013): 125-33. doi:10.1177/2042098613482484

21. Malchodi L, Wagner K, Susi A, et al. Early acid suppression therapy exposure and fracture in young children. *Pediatrics.* 2019; 144(1); pii:e20182625; doi: 10.1542/peds.2018-262

22. Trikha, Anita et al. Development of food allergies in patients with gastroesophageal reflux disease treated with gastric acid suppressive medications. *Pediatric Allergy and Immunology: official publication of the*

European Society of Pediatric Allergy and Immunology vol. 24,6 (2013): 582-8. doi:10.1111/pai.12103

Chapter 4: How feeding and baby care affect reflux

1. Bergman NJ. Neonatal stomach volume and physiology suggest feeding at 1-h intervals. *Acta Paediatr.* 2013;102(8):773-777. doi:10.1111/apa.12291

2. Prime DK, Geddes DT, Hartmann PE. Oxytocin: milk ejection and maternal-infant well-being. In: Hale T, Hartmann PE, editors. *Textbook of Human Lactation.* 1st ed. Amarillo: Hale Publishing; 2007. p. 141–58

3. APA Dudek-Shriber, Linda EdD, OTR/L; Zelazny, Susan MS, OTR/L The Effects of Prone Positioning on the Quality and Acquisition of Developmental Milestones in Four-Month-Old Infants. *Pediatric Physical Therapy*: April 2007, Volume 19, Issue 1, p48-55 doi: 10.1097/01.pep.0000234963.72945.b1

4. Chang YJ, Anderson GC, Lin CH. Effects of prone and supine positions on sleep state and stress responses in mechanically ventilated preterm infants during the first postnatal week. *J Adv Nurs.* 2002;40(2):161-169. doi:10.1046/j.1365-2648.2002.02358.x

5. Bergman, N. Proposal for mechanisms of protection of supine sleep against sudden infant death syndrome: an integrated mechanism review. *Pediatr Res* 77, 10–19 (2015). https://doi.org/10.1038/pr.2014.140

6. Majnemer A, Barr RG. Influence of supine sleep positioning on early motor milestone acquisition. *Dev Med Child Neurol.* 2005;47(6):370-364. doi:10.1017/s0012162205000733

7. Robertson, R. Supine infant positioning - Yes, but there's more to it. *J Fam Pract.* 2011 October;60(10):605-608

8. Dudek-Shriber, Linda EdD, OTR/L; Zelazny, Susan MS, OTR/L The Effects of Prone Positioning on the Quality and Acquisition of Developmental Milestones in Four-Month-Old Infants. *Pediatric Physical Therapy*: April 2007, Volume 19, Issue 1, p48-55 doi: 10.1097/01.pep.0000234963.72945.b1

9. Luigi Corvaglia, Raffaella Rotatori, Marianna Ferlini, Arianna Aceti, Gina Ancora, Giacomo Faldella. The Effect of Body Positioning on Gastroesophageal Reflux in Premature Infants: Evaluation by Combined Impedance and pH Monitoring. *The Journal of Pediatrics*, Volume 151, Issue 6, 2007, Pages 591-596.e1, doi:10.1016/j.jpeds.2007.06.014.

10. Kuo P, Bravi I, Marreddy U, Aziz Q, Sifrim D. Postprandial cardiac vagal tone and transient lower esophageal sphincter relaxation (TLESR). *Neurogastroenterol Motil.* 2013;25(10):841-e639. doi:10.1111/nmo.12195

11. Tougas, G et al. Cardiac autonomic function and oesophageal acid sensitivity in patients with non-cardiac chest pain. *Gut* vol. 49,5 (2001): 706-12. doi:10.1136/gut.49.5.706

12. http://www.kangaroomothercare.com/1new-page.aspx

13. Barr RG, Konner M, Bakeman R, Adamson L. Crying in !Kung San infants: a test of the cultural specificity hypothesis. *Dev Med Child Neurol.* 1991;33(7):601-610. doi:10.1111/j.1469-8749.1991.tb14930.x

14. James-Roberts, Ian & Alvarez, Marissa & Csipke, Emese & Abramsky, Tanya & Goodwin, Jennifer & Sorgenfrei, Esther. (2006). Infant Crying and Sleeping in London, Copenhagen and When Parents Adopt a 'Proximal' Form of Care. *Pediatrics* 2006;117;e1146 DOI: 10.1542/peds.2005-2387. Pediatrics. 117. e1146-55. 10.1542/peds.2005-2387.

15. Kaur R, Bharti B, Saini SK. A randomized controlled trial of burping for the prevention of colic and regurgitation in healthy infants. *Child Care Health Dev.* 2015;41(1):52-56. doi:10.1111/cch.12166

16. Orenstein, S., (1990). Prone positioning in infant gastroesophageal reflux: Is elevation of the head worth the trouble? *J Pediatr* 117:2, part 1. 184-187.

17. Tobin JM, McCloud P, Cameron DJS Posture and gastro-oesophageal reflux: a case for left lateral positioning. *Archives of Disease in Childhood* 1997;76:254-258.

18. Vandenplas, Yvan; Rudolph, Colin D; Di Lorenzo, Carlo; Hassall, Eric; Liptak, Gregory; Mazur, Lynnette; Sondheimer, Judith; Staiano, Annamaria; Thomson, Michael; Veereman-Wauters, Gigi; Wenzl, Tobias G Co-Chairs:Committee Members: Pediatric Gastroesophageal Reflux Clinical Practice Guidelines: Joint Recommendations of the North American Society for Pediatric Gastroenterology, Hepatology, and Nutrition (NASPGHAN) and the European Society for Pediatric Gastroenterology, Hepatology, and Nutrition (ESPGHAN). *Journal of Pediatric Gastroenterology and Nutrition:* October 2009, Volume 49, Issue 4, p498-547 doi: 10.1097/MPG.0b013e3181b7f563

19. Kahn, A., Rebuffat, E., Sottiaux, M. et al. Lack of temporal relation between acid reflux in the proximal oesophagus and cardiorespiratory events in sleeping infants. *Eur J Pediatr* 151, 208–212 (1992). https://doi.org/10.1007/BF01954386

20. Morgan BE, Horn AR, Bergman NJ. Should neonates sleep alone? *Biol Psychiatry.* 2011;70(9):817-825. doi:10.1016/j.biopsych.2011.06.018

21. Heacock, Helen J.; Jeffery, Heather E.; Baker, Jennifer L.; Page, Megan. Influence of Breast Versus Formula Milk on Physiological Gastroesophageal Reflux in Healthy, Newborn Infants *Journal of Pediatric Gastroenterology and Nutrition.* 14(1):41-46, January 1992

22. Campanozzi A, Boccia G, Pensabene L, et al. Prevalence and natural history of gastroesophageal reflux: pediatric prospective survey. *Pediatrics.* 2009;123(3):779-783. doi:10.1542/peds.2007-3569

23. De Giorgi, F et al. Pathophysiology of gastro-oesophageal reflux disease. *Acta otorhinolaryngologica Italica*: organo ufficiale della Societa italiana

di otorinolaringologia e chirurgia cervico-facciale vol. 26,5 (2006): 241-6.

24. Hale, Thomas & Rowe, Hilary. *Medications & Mother's Milk*. Springer Publishing Company, New York 2017

25. Pehl C, Pfeiffer A, Wendl B, Kaess H. The effect of decaffeination of coffee on gastro-oesophageal reflux in patients with reflux disease. *Aliment Pharmacol Ther*. 1997;11(3):483-486. doi:10.1046/j.1365-2036.1997.00161.x

26. Mohrbacher, Nancy. *Breastfeeding Answers Made Simple*. Hale Publishing 2010

Chapter 5: Exploring reflux symptoms - are they always reflux?

1. Steger M., Schneemann M, Fox M. Systematic review: the pathogenesis and pharmacological treatment of hiccups. *Alimentary Pharmacology and Therapeutics*. 2015; Vol 42, Issue 9

2. Brouillette RT, Thach BT, Abu-Osba YK, Wilson SL. Hiccups in infants: characteristics and effects on ventilation. *J Pediatr*. 1980 Feb;96(2):219-25. doi: 10.1016/s0022-3476(80)80806-7. PMID: 7351583.

3. Whitehead, K., Jones, L., Laudiano-Dray, M.P., Meek, J. & Fabrizi, L. Event-related potentials following contraction of respiratory muscles in pre-term and full-term infants. *Clin. Neurophysiol*. 130, 2216–2221 (2019)

4. Messner AH, Lalakea ML, Aby J, Macmahon J, Bair E. Ankyloglossia: incidence and associated feeding difficulties. *Arch Otolaryngol Head Neck Surg*. 2000;126(1):36-39. doi:10.1001/archotol.126.1.36

5. Rubio, Amandine & Griffet, Jacques & Caci, Hervé & Bérard, Etienne & Hayek, Toni & Boutté, Patrick. (2008). The moulded baby syndrome: Incidence and risk factors regarding 1,001 neonates. *European Journal of Pediatrics*. 168. 605-11. 10.1007/s00431-008-0806-y.

6. Lucassen, P L et al. Systematic review of the occurrence of infantile colic in the community. *Archives of Disease in Childhood* vol. 84,5 (2001): 398-403. doi:10.1136/adc.84.5.398

7. Stern E, Parmelee AH, Akiyama Y, Schultz MA, Wenner WH. Sleep cycle characteristics in infants. *Pediatrics*. 1969;43(1):65-70.

8. Henderson JM, France KG, Owens JL, Blampied NM. Sleeping through the night: the consolidation of self-regulated sleep across the first year of life. *Pediatrics*. 2010;126(5):e1081-e1087. doi:10.1542/peds.2010-0976

9. Drake C, Roehrs T, Shambroom J, Roth T. Caffeine effects on sleep taken 0, 3, or 6 hours before going to bed. *J Clin Sleep Med*. 2013;9(11):1195-1200. Published 2013 Nov 15. doi:10.5664/jcsm.3170

10. Sender R, Fuchs S, Milo R. Revised Estimates for the Number of Human and Bacteria Cells in the Body. *PLoS Biol*. 2016;14(8):e1002533. Pub-

lished 2016 Aug 19. doi:10.1371/journal.pbio.1002533

11. https://badgut.org/information-centre/a-z-digestive-topics/intestinal-gas/

12. Pamela Douglas, Donna Geddes. Practice-based interpretation of ultrasound studies leads the way to more effective clinical support and less pharmaceutical and surgical intervention for breastfeeding infants. *Midwifery*, Volume 58. 2018 Pages 145-155, ISSN 0266-6138, doi:10.1016/j.midw.2017.12.007.

13. Ludington-Hoe SM, Cong X, Hashemi F. Infant crying: nature, physiologic consequences, and select interventions. *Neonatal Netw*. 2002;21(2):29-36. doi:10.1891/0730-0832.21.2.29

14. Werlin SL, Dodds WJ, Hogan WJ, Arndorfer RC. Mechanisms of gastroesophageal reflux in children. *J Pediatr*. 1980;97(2):244-249. doi:10.1016/s0022-3476(80)80482-3

15. Gabriella Boccia, Roberta Buonavolontà, Paola Coccorullo, Francesco Manguso, Laura Fuiano, Annamaria Staiano, Dyspeptic Symptoms in Children: The Result of a Constipation-Induced Cologastric Brake? *Clinical Gastroenterology and Hepatology*, Volume 6, Issue 5, 2008, Pages 556-560, ISSN 1542-3565 https://doi.org/10.1016/j.cgh.2008.01.001.

16. Borowitz S.M. Sutphen J.L. Recurrent vomiting and persistent gastroesophageal reflux caused by unrecognized constipation. *Clin Pediatr*. 2004; 43: 461-466

17. A. Marcobal, J. L. Sonnenburg 2013 Human milk oligosaccharide consumption by intestinal microbiota. *Clin Microbiol Infect*. 2012 Jul; 18(0 4): 12–15.

18. Palmer, Linda F. *Baby Poop: What your Paediatrician may not tell you*. Sunny Lane Press, 2015

Chapter 6: Your baby and reflux

1. Walker, M. *Breastfeeding Management for the Clinician*, Jones & Bartlett Publishers, 2013

2. Mohrbacher, N. *Breastfeeding Answers Made Simple*. Hale Publishing 2010

3. Uvnäs-Moberg, Kerstin, Widstrom, Ann-marie, Marchini, Giovanna and Winberg, Jan (2008). Release of GI Hormones in Mother and Infant by Sensory Stimulation. *Acta Paediatrica*. 76. 851 - 860. 10.1111/j.1651-2227.1987.tb17254.x.

4. Boccia G, Buonavolontà R, Coccorullo P, Manguso F, Fuiano L, Staiano A. Dyspeptic symptoms in children: the result of a constipation-induced cologastric brake? *Clin Gastroenterol Hepatol*. 2008;6(5):556-560. doi:10.1016/j.cgh.2008.01.001.

Chapter 7: Strategies and techniques

1. Disantis KI, Collins BN, Fisher JO, Davey A. Do infants fed directly from the breast have improved appetite regulation and slower growth during early childhood compared with infants fed from a bottle?. *Int J Behav Nutr Phys Act.* 2011;8:89. Published 2011 Aug 17. doi:10.1186/1479-5868-8-89

2. Li, Ruowei & Magadia, Joselito & Grummer-Strawn, Laurence. (2012). Risk of Bottle-feeding for Rapid Weight Gain During the First Year of Life. *Archives of Pediatrics & Adolescent Medicine.* 166. 431-6. 10.1001/archpediatrics.2011.1665

3. Li, Ruowei & Scanlon, Kelley & May, Ashleigh & Rose, Chelsea & Birch, Leann. (2014). Bottle-Feeding Practices During Early Infancy and Eating Behaviors at 6 Years of Age. *Pediatrics.* 134 Suppl 1. S70-7. 10.1542/peds.2014-0646L.

4. Kramer MS, Guo T, Platt RW, et al. Feeding effects on growth during infancy. *J Pediatr.* 2004;145(5):600-605. doi:10.1016/j.jpeds.2004.06.069

5. Hunziker UA, Barr RG. Increased carrying reduces infant crying: a randomized controlled trial. *Pediatrics.* 1986;77(5):641-648.

6. Frank A. Scafidi, Tiffany M. Field, Saul M. Schanberg, Charles R. Bauer, Karen Tucci, Jacqueline Roberts, Connie Morrow, Cynthia M. Kuhn, Massage stimulates growth in preterm infants: A replication. *Infant Behavior and Development,* Volume 13, Issue 2, 1990, Pages 167-188, ISSN 0163-6383. doi.org:10.1016/0163-6383(90)90029-8

7. Ball, H. Parent-infant bed-sharing behavior. *Hum Nat* 17, 301–318 (2006). doi:10.1007/s12110-006-1011-1

8. Dahlen, Hannah Grace et al. Gastro-oesophageal reflux: a mixed methods study of infants admitted to hospital in the first 12 months following birth in NSW (2000-2011). *BMC Pediatrics* vol. 18,1 30. 12 Feb. 2018, doi:10.1186/s12887-018-0999-9

9. Minchin, M. *Crying babies and food in the early years.* Alma Publications, 2016.

Chapter 8: Beyond reflux – co-regulating your baby

1. https://bcscw.wildapricot.org/Resources/Documents/bergman1.pdf

2. Bergman, N.J., 2014, 'The neuroscience of birth – and the case for Zero Separation', Curationis 37(2), Art. #1440,4 page. http://dx.doi.org/10.4102/curationis.v37i2.1440

3. Hofer, M.A. The psychobiology of early attachment. *Clinical Neuroscience Research* 4(5–6), 291–300. (2005) http://dx.doi.org/10.1016/j.cnr.2005.03.007

4. Barr RG, Konner M, Bakeman R, Adamson L. Crying in !Kung San infants: a test of the cultural specificity hypothesis. *Dev Med Child Neurol.*

1991;33(7):601-610. doi:10.1111/j.1469-8749.1991.tb14930.x

5. James-Roberts, Ian, Alvarez, Marissa, Csipke, Emese, Abramsky, Tanya, Goodwin, Jennifer and Sorgenfrei, Esther (2006). Infant Crying and Sleeping in London, Copenhagen and When Parents Adopt a 'Proximal' Form of Care. *Pediatrics* 2006;117;e1146 DOI: 10.1542/peds.2005-2387.

6. Morgan BE, Horn AR, Bergman NJ. Should neonates sleep alone?. *Biol Psychiatry*. 2011;70(9):817-825. doi:10.1016/j.biopsych.2011.06.018

7. Henderson JM, France KG, Owens JL, Blampied NM. Sleeping through the night: the consolidation of self-regulated sleep across the first year of life. *Pediatrics*. 2010;126(5):e1081-e1087. doi:10.1542/peds.2010-0976

8. H.L. Ball (2002) Reasons to bed-share: Why parents sleep with their infants. *Journal of Reproductive and Infant Psychology*, 20:4, 207-221, DOI: 10.1080/0264683021000033147

9. Fern R. Hauck, Kawai O. Tanabe. International Trends in Sudden Infant Death Syndrome: Stabilization of Rates Requires Further Action. *Pediatrics* Sep 2008, 122 (3) 660-666; DOI: 10.1542/peds.2007-0135

10. S. Mosko, C. Richard, J. McKenna, Maternal Sleep and Arousals During Bedsharing With Infants, *Sleep*, Volume 20, Issue 2, February 1997, Pages 142–150, https://doi.org/10.1093/sleep/20.2.142

11. Stephen W. Porges. The polyvagal theory: phylogenetic substrates of a social nervous system. *International Journal of Psychophysiology*, Volume 42, Issue 2, 2001, p123-146, ISSN 0167-8760, https://doi.org/10.1016/S0167-8760(01)00162-3

12. Alvarez M. Caregiving and Early Infant Crying in a Danish Community. *Developmental and Behavioral Pediatrics*. 2004;25(2):91-8.

13. Lucassen, P L et al. Systematic review of the occurrence of infantile colic in the community. *Archives of Disease in Childhood* vol. 84,5 (2001): 398-403. doi:10.1136/adc.84.5.398

14. McKenna, J.J, Middlemiss, W., Tarsha, M.S. Potential Evolutionary, Neurophysiological, and Developmental Origins of Sudden Infant Death Syndrome and Inconsolable Crying (Colic): Is It About Controlling Breath? *Family Relations* Volume 65, Issue1 Special Issue on Biosocial Models of Family Science, February 2016, p239-258 https://doi.org/10.1111/fare.12178

15. Grille, Robin. *Heart to Heart Parenting*. Australian Broadcasting Commission, 2008

16. Almanza-Sepulveda ML, Fleming AS, Jonas W. Mothering revisited: A role for cortisol? *Hormones and Behavior*. 2020 May;121:104679. DOI: 10.1016/j.yhbeh.2020.104679.

17. Tronick, E. and A.F. Gianino. Interactive mismatch and repair: Challenges to the coping infant. *Zero to Three* 6(3) (1986): 1-6.

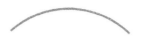

Index

Available from Pinter & Martin
in the **Why it Matters** *series*

Series editor: Susan Last

pinterandmartin.com

Printed in the USA
CPSIA information can be obtained
at www.ICGtesting.com
JSHW012053140824
68134JS00035B/3408